AF367063

Breast Cancer

-

From Causes to Control

by

VIRUTI SHIVAN

Masters in Clinical Psychology (Major)

"In books, as in life, it's not the size or looks but the content that matters."

Introduction

Breast cancer is a journey that begins long before diagnosis and extends far beyond treatment. This book is designed to be your companion through every step of that journey, from the first whisper of concern through the complex decisions about treatment and into the world of post-cancer life. Our aim is not only to inform but to empower, offering a source of strength, knowledge, and hope for those affected by breast cancer and their loved ones.

Breast Cancer: A Complex Enemy

At its core, breast cancer is not a single disease but a spectrum of conditions characterized by the uncontrolled growth of breast cells. The complexity of breast cancer lies not only in its biological underpinnings but also in the deeply personal stories of those it touches. Each person's experience with breast cancer is unique, influenced by their biology, their environment, and their life circumstances. It's a disease that challenges not just the body but the spirit, demanding resilience, courage, and a profound sense of hope.

Knowledge as Power

Knowledge is your greatest ally in the fight against breast cancer. Understanding the enemy — its causes, its mechanisms, and its weaknesses — is the first step toward victory. This book will guide you through the scientific landscape of breast cancer, demystifying terms, explaining concepts, and illuminating pathways through the maze of treatment options. But beyond the science, this book also seeks to understand the human experience of breast cancer, exploring the emotional, psychological, and social challenges that accompany a diagnosis.

Empowerment through Understanding

Empowerment comes from understanding not just the disease but also the broader context in which it exists. This includes recognizing the role of lifestyle factors, the importance of early detection, and the power of an informed, proactive approach to health. It also means navigating the healthcare system, understanding your rights and options, and learning how to advocate for yourself and others. This book aims to equip you with the tools you need to take control of your health and to face breast cancer with confidence and determination.

A Guide for the Journey

This book is structured to reflect the journey through breast cancer, from the initial diagnosis to the challenges of treatment and the questions that arise in its aftermath. It includes insights into the latest research and emerging treatments, offering a glimpse into the future of breast cancer care. But it also emphasizes the timeless elements of the human experience — the strength found in community, the healing power of empathy, and the enduring hope that guides us through the darkest times.

As we embark on this journey together, remember that you are not alone. Thousands of others have walked this path before you, armed with determination and guided by hope. This book is a testament to their strength and a tool for your own journey. With each page, may you find not only information but also inspiration, not just facts but also faith. Welcome to your comprehensive guide to breast cancer, from causes to control.

Chapter 1: Understanding Breast Cancer

1.1 The Basics of Breast Cancer

Breast cancer, at its most fundamental level, is a malignancy that develops in the cells of the breasts. This disease can affect both men and women, but it is far more common in women, significantly impacting millions of lives around the globe each year. Understanding the basics of breast cancer is the first step toward empowerment, enabling individuals to navigate the journey that lies ahead with knowledge and confidence.

What is Breast Cancer?

Breast cancer begins when cells in the breast grow uncontrollably, forming a tumor that can often be seen on an x-ray or felt as a lump. These cancerous cells can spread (metastasize) to other parts of the body, making early detection and treatment crucial to improving outcomes. The disease is not monolithic; it comprises several types, including hormone receptor-positive, HER2-positive, and triple-negative breast cancers, each with distinct characteristics and treatment responses.

Causes and Risk Factors

While the exact cause of breast cancer remains unknown, several risk factors have been identified. These include genetic mutations (such as BRCA1 and BRCA2), family history of the disease, age, dense breast tissue, exposure to estrogen, lifestyle factors (such as alcohol consumption, obesity, and physical inactivity), and reproductive history. It's important to note that having one or even several risk factors does not mean an individual will definitely develop breast cancer; however, understanding these risks can guide preventive measures and screening practices.

Symptoms of Breast Cancer

Breast cancer symptoms vary widely – from no symptoms at all to noticeable changes in the breast. Common signs include a lump or thickening in the breast or underarm, changes to the size or shape of the breast, dimpling or irritation of breast skin, redness or flaky skin in the nipple area or the breast, pulling in of the nipple or pain in the nipple area, and nipple discharge other than breast milk, including blood. Not all lumps or alterations are cancerous, but any persistent change should be evaluated by a healthcare professional.

Importance of Screening

Screening for breast cancer primarily involves mammography, an x-ray exam of the breast used to detect and evaluate breast changes. Early detection through regular screening can significantly increase the chances of successful treatment, emphasizing the importance of awareness and proactive health management. Guidelines on screening vary, but they generally recommend that women of average risk begin mammograms at a certain age and continue them at regular intervals.

The Path Forward

Understanding the basics of breast cancer lays the groundwork for a deeper exploration of its complexities. Knowledge of the disease's nature, risk factors, and the paramount importance of early detection provides a solid foundation upon which individuals can build a proactive approach to their health, armed with the information necessary to navigate the challenges of diagnosis, treatment, and beyond. As we move forward, remember that knowledge is power, and empowerment begins with understanding.

1.2 Risk Factors and Prevention

Identifying and understanding the risk factors for breast cancer are crucial steps in managing and potentially reducing one's risk of developing the disease. While some factors, such as age or genetics, are beyond our control, there are lifestyle choices and preventive measures that can significantly influence the risk.

Non-Modifiable Risk Factors

- **Genetic Mutations**: Certain inherited genetic mutations, most notably BRCA1 and BRCA2, significantly increase the risk of breast and ovarian cancers.

- **Family History**: Having a close relative with breast cancer doubles one's risk. The risk increases further if multiple family members are affected or if a family member was diagnosed at a young age.

- **Age**: The risk of developing breast cancer increases with age. Most breast cancers are diagnosed after age 50.

- **Dense Breast Tissue**: Women with dense breasts have a higher risk of breast cancer. Dense breast tissue can also make mammograms less effective in detecting tumors.

Modifiable Risk Factors

- **Lifestyle Choices**: Diet, physical activity, and alcohol consumption can influence breast cancer risk. Maintaining a healthy weight, engaging in regular physical activity, and limiting alcohol intake are recommended.

- **Reproductive History**: Early menstruation (before age 12), late menopause (after age 55), having your first child at an older age, or never having given birth can increase breast cancer risk.

- **Hormone Replacement Therapy (HRT)**: Long-term use of hormone replacement therapy, especially combined estrogen and progestin, has been linked to an increased risk of breast cancer.

Prevention Strategies

- **Regular Screening**: Early detection through mammograms can save lives, allowing for treatment before the cancer spreads.

- **Lifestyle Modifications**: Adopting a healthy lifestyle by eating a balanced diet rich in fruits and vegetables, staying physically active, and maintaining a healthy weight can help reduce the risk of breast cancer.

- **Limit Alcohol Consumption**: Limiting alcohol to no more than one drink per day may help reduce breast cancer risk.

- **Breastfeeding**: Breastfeeding for a total of one year or more (for all children) can lower the risk of breast cancer.

- **Avoiding Exposure to Radiation and Environmental Pollution**: Limiting exposure to radiations from medical imaging tests like CT scans and reducing exposure to endocrine disruptors and carcinogens found in some plastics and cosmetics can be beneficial.

Chemoprevention and Surgical Options

For women at high risk of breast cancer, medications like tamoxifen and raloxifene have been shown to reduce risk. In very high-risk scenarios, prophylactic surgeries, such as mastectomy and oophorectomy, have been considered and undertaken to significantly lower the risk of breast cancer.

Understanding the complex interplay of risk factors for breast cancer allows individuals to make informed decisions about their health. While not all risk factors are within our control, awareness and proactive management of those that are modifiable can empower women to take charge of their breast health.

1.3 Symptoms and Early Detection

The early detection of breast cancer significantly improves the prognosis and increases the likelihood of successful treatment. Recognizing the symptoms of breast cancer and understanding the importance of early detection are crucial steps in the fight against this disease.

Symptoms of Breast Cancer

Early breast cancer often does not cause symptoms. However, as the tumor grows, it can change how the breast looks or feels. The common symptoms include:

- **Lump or Thickening**: A new lump or thickening in the breast or underarm area, distinct from the other breast tissue.

- **Change in Size, Shape, or Appearance**: Any change in the size, shape, or appearance of the breast or nipple.

- **Skin Changes**: Dimpling, puckering, scaling, or redness of the breast skin that can resemble an orange peel.

- **Nipple Changes**: Turning inward of the nipple, redness, scaling, or a nipple discharge other than breast milk, particularly if it's bloody.

- **Pain**: Although lumps are often painless, pain or tenderness in the breast can be a symptom of breast cancer.

It's important to note that these symptoms can also be caused by conditions other than breast cancer. However, any persistent changes should be evaluated by a healthcare professional.

Early Detection Strategies

- **Breast Self-Exams (BSE)**: While breast self-exams are not a substitute for mammograms or clinical exams, becoming familiar with the normal appearance and feel of your breasts may help you notice changes or abnormalities. If you detect any, report them to your doctor promptly.

- **Clinical Breast Exams (CBE)**: A clinical breast exam performed by a healthcare professional should be part of a periodic health exam, about every three years for women in their 20s and 30s and every year for women 40 and over.

- **Mammography**: Mammograms are the most effective screening tool used to find breast cancer before it causes symptoms. Women aged 40 to 44 should have the option to start annual breast cancer screening with mammograms if they wish to do so. Women 45 to 54 should get mammograms every year. Women 55 and older can switch to mammograms every 2 years, or continue yearly screening.

The Role of Genetic Testing and MRI

For women at high risk of breast cancer, additional tests may be recommended:

- **Genetic Testing**: For those with a family history of breast or ovarian cancer, genetic testing can identify specific mutations in genes (like BRCA1 or BRCA2) that increase the risk of breast cancer.

- **Breast MRI**: MRI is used along with mammograms for screening women at high risk of breast cancer. It is not used for women at average risk because it may find cancers that are not there (false positives), leading to unnecessary tests and anxiety.

Conclusion

Recognizing the symptoms and understanding the importance of early detection are key in the fight against breast cancer. Regular screening and prompt attention to changes in the breast can lead to early diagnosis, when the disease is most treatable. Talk to your healthcare provider about your risk of breast cancer and the best screening plan for you. Remember, early detection saves lives.

1.4 Exercise: 10 MCQs with Answers at the End

Below are 10 multiple-choice questions (MCQs) designed to test your understanding of breast cancer basics, risk factors, prevention, symptoms, and early detection. Answers are provided at the end to help you assess your knowledge.

1. What is the most common type of breast cancer?

   A. Invasive ductal carcinoma

   B. Lobular carcinoma in situ

   C. Invasive lobular carcinoma

   D. Ductal carcinoma in situ

2. Which gene mutation is most commonly associated with a higher risk of breast cancer?

   A. BRCA1

   B. TP53

   C. MYC

   D. RB1

3. At what age is it recommended for women of average risk to start having mammograms every year?

   A. 40

B. 45

C. 50

D. 55

4. Which of the following is NOT a known risk factor for breast cancer?

A. High-fat diet

B. Alcohol consumption

C. Physical inactivity

D. Frequent use of antiperspirants

5. What is a common early symptom of breast cancer?

A. High fever

B. Severe breast pain

C. A new lump in the breast or underarm

D. Sudden weight gain

6. Which lifestyle change can help reduce the risk of breast cancer?

A. Increasing alcohol consumption

B. Gaining weight

C. Staying physically active

D. Using hormone replacement therapy

7. What is the purpose of breast self-exams (BSE)?

   A. To definitely determine if a lump is cancerous

   B. To replace mammography screening

   C. To become familiar with the normal look and feel of one's breasts

   D. To decrease the need for clinical breast exams

8. How can dense breast tissue affect breast cancer screening?

   A. Makes it easier to detect tumors with a mammogram

   B. Reduces the need for additional screening

   C. Can make mammograms less effective at detecting tumors

   D. Increases the accuracy of ultrasound screenings only

9. What is the benefit of genetic testing for individuals with a family history of breast cancer?

   A. It can predict with certainty who will develop breast cancer

   B. It eliminates the need for regular breast cancer screening

   C. It identifies specific genetic mutations that increase the risk of breast cancer

   D. It can determine the best dietary changes to prevent breast cancer

10. Which preventive measure is recommended for women at high risk of breast cancer?

   A. Avoiding all screenings to reduce stress

   B. Prophylactic mastectomy

   C. Never using birth control pills

   D. Consuming a high-fat diet

Answers:

1. A. Invasive ductal carcinoma

2. A. BRCA1

3. B. 45

4. D. Frequent use of antiperspirants

5. C. A new lump in the breast or underarm

6. C. Staying physically active

7. C. To become familiar with the normal look and feel of one's breasts

8. C. Can make mammograms less effective at detecting tumors

9. C. It identifies specific genetic mutations that increase the risk of breast cancer

10. B. Prophylactic mastectomy

Chapter 2: The Diagnosis Journey

2.1 Screening Methods and Their Importance

The journey to diagnosing breast cancer often begins with screening methods designed to detect cancer before symptoms appear. These early detection strategies are crucial for improving the prognosis and increasing the survival rates of those diagnosed with breast cancer. Here, we delve into the primary screening methods and their significance in the early detection and management of breast cancer.

Mammography

The cornerstone of breast cancer screening is mammography, an X-ray technique specifically designed to visualize the breast tissue. Mammograms can detect tumors that are too small to be felt and can identify suspicious areas that may require further testing. There are two main types of mammograms:

- **Screening Mammogram**: Used routinely to check for breast cancer in women who have no symptoms.

- **Diagnostic Mammogram**: Used to investigate suspicious breast changes, such as a new breast lump, pain, or nipple discharge that has been noticed by the patient or on a screening mammogram.

Breast Magnetic Resonance Imaging (MRI)

Breast MRI is a more sensitive imaging technique than mammography and is used in conjunction with mammograms for high-risk individuals. It uses magnetic fields and radio waves to create detailed images of the breast. MRI is particularly beneficial for screening women with a high risk of breast cancer due to genetic factors, family history, or other specific conditions.

Ultrasound

Breast ultrasound utilizes sound waves to produce images of the internal structures of the breast. It is often used as a complementary tool to mammography, especially in women with dense breast tissue where mammograms may be less effective. Ultrasound can help distinguish between solid masses (which are more likely to be cancerous) and fluid-filled cysts (which are less likely to be cancerous).

Clinical Breast Exam (CBE)

A clinical breast exam is performed by a healthcare professional who uses their hands to feel for lumps or other changes in the breast and underarm area. Though not a primary screening tool for breast cancer, CBE can be an important component of a comprehensive breast health evaluation, particularly for women who have symptoms of breast cancer.

The Importance of Screening

Early detection through regular screening is vital for catching breast cancer at an early stage, when it is most treatable. The goal of screening is not only to detect cancer early but also to reduce the chance of mortality through timely and effective intervention. While screening does not prevent breast cancer, it can significantly reduce the risk of death from the disease by finding cancers when they are more likely to be small, less likely to have spread, and more responsive to treatment.

Screening guidelines vary based on factors such as age, family history, and risk level. It is essential for individuals to discuss their personal risk factors with a healthcare provider to determine the most appropriate screening schedule for their specific situation.

Conclusion

Screening plays a pivotal role in the early detection of breast cancer, offering a critical window for intervention before the disease progresses. Understanding and utilizing the appropriate screening methods are key components of effective breast cancer management and care. By prioritizing regular screenings, individuals can take proactive steps towards safeguarding their health and improving their chances of successful treatment outcomes.

2.2 Biopsy and Diagnosis

After a suspicious area is detected through breast cancer screening, the next step in the diagnosis journey is often a biopsy. A biopsy is the only definitive way to diagnose breast cancer, as it involves the removal of cells or tissue from the suspicious area for examination under a microscope by a pathologist. This section explores the various types of biopsies used in diagnosing breast cancer and the process leading to a definitive diagnosis.

Types of Biopsies

- **Fine Needle Aspiration Biopsy (FNAB)**: This minimally invasive procedure uses a thin, hollow needle to remove a small amount of cells from the suspicious area. FNAB can help determine if a lump is solid or filled with fluid.

- **Core Needle Biopsy (CNB)**: A larger needle is used in CNB to remove a small cylinder of tissue, providing more detailed information than FNAB. This method is preferred when cancer is suspected because it can provide enough tissue for a definitive diagnosis without the need for surgery.

- **Stereotactic Biopsy**: This technique is used primarily for abnormalities seen on a mammogram that cannot be felt. Using computer-guided imagery, a needle is precisely directed to the area of concern to collect tissue samples.

- **Ultrasound-Guided Biopsy**: When an abnormality is visible on an ultrasound, this type of biopsy uses ultrasound imaging to guide the needle to the correct location.

- **MRI-Guided Biopsy**: For abnormalities that are best seen on MRI, this biopsy is performed with the help of MRI guidance to ensure accurate sampling of the suspicious area.

- **Surgical (Open) Biopsy**: In some cases, a surgical biopsy may be necessary. This involves the removal of part (incisional biopsy) or all (excisional biopsy) of the lump for examination. Surgical biopsies are less common for initial diagnosis due to the effectiveness of less invasive methods.

The Diagnosis Process

After the biopsy, the collected samples are analyzed by a pathologist who checks for cancer cells. The pathology report includes details about the type of cancer, grade (how much cancer cells resemble healthy cells, indicating how quickly the cells are likely to grow and spread), and receptor status (such as estrogen receptor, progesterone receptor, and HER2/neu status). This information is crucial for determining the most effective treatment plan.

Additional Diagnostic Tests

Following a positive biopsy result, additional tests may be recommended to understand the extent of cancer and whether it has spread. These can include:

- **Blood Tests**: To check for markers that indicate cancer.

- **Imaging Tests**: Such as bone scans, chest X-rays, CT scans, and PET scans to look for signs of cancer spread.

The Importance of a Multidisciplinary Approach

A diagnosis of breast cancer typically involves a team of specialists, including a radiologist, pathologist, surgeon, oncologist, and possibly others. This multidisciplinary approach ensures that every aspect of the diagnosis and treatment plan is carefully considered, providing comprehensive care to the patient.

Conclusion

Biopsy and subsequent diagnosis are critical steps in the journey of a breast cancer patient, offering the definitive answer needed to proceed with treatment. Understanding the types of biopsies and the diagnostic process helps patients navigate their care with knowledge and confidence, empowering them to make informed decisions about their treatment options.

2.3 Interpreting Your Pathology Report

After undergoing a biopsy to investigate a suspicious area in the breast, the next critical step in the diagnosis journey is interpreting the pathology report. This document is a detailed account provided by a pathologist after examining the biopsy samples under a microscope. It contains vital information about the presence or absence of cancer, the type of cancer, and its characteristics. Understanding your pathology report is essential for making informed decisions about your treatment options.

Key Components of a Pathology Report

- **Patient and Specimen Information**: This section includes identifying information about the patient and details about the biopsy specimen, such as when and where the biopsy was performed.

- **Diagnosis**: The diagnosis section is the heart of the report. It indicates whether cancer cells were found in the sample. If cancer is present, this section will detail the type of breast cancer (e.g., invasive ductal carcinoma, ductal carcinoma in situ) and the tumor grade.

- **Tumor Grade**: The grade describes how much the cancer cells resemble normal breast cells and suggests how quickly the cancer is likely to grow and spread. It is usually expressed on a scale of 1 to 3, with Grade 1 being well-differentiated (slow-growing) and Grade 3 being poorly differentiated (fast-growing).

- **Tumor Size**: This measurement is critical for staging the cancer and determining the treatment plan. It is often reported in millimeters (mm) or centimeters (cm).

- **Margins**: The margins indicate whether cancer cells were found at the edge of the biopsy sample. "Clear" or "negative" margins mean no cancer cells are at the edges, suggesting that the cancer was likely removed completely. "Positive" margins indicate that cancer cells are present at the edge, suggesting that some cancer might still be in the breast.

- **Lymph Node Status**: If a lymph node biopsy was performed, this section provides information about whether cancer cells were found in the lymph nodes, which can indicate whether the cancer has begun to spread.

- **Hormone Receptor Status**: This part of the report indicates whether the cancer cells have receptors for estrogen (ER) and/or progesterone (PR). Cancers that are hormone receptor-positive can often be treated with hormone therapy.

- **HER2/neu Status**: The report will also indicate whether the cancer cells produce an excess of the HER2 protein. HER2-positive cancers may be treated with drugs that specifically target this protein.

- **Conclusion**: The conclusion summarizes the key findings of the pathology report. It is a concise overview of the diagnosis and the characteristics of the cancer.

The Role of the Pathology Report in Treatment Planning

The details in the pathology report play a crucial role in determining the most appropriate treatment plan for breast cancer. Factors such as the type of cancer, tumor grade, hormone receptor status, and HER2 status can influence the choice of surgery, the need for chemotherapy, radiation therapy, hormone therapy, and targeted therapy options.

Communicating with Your Healthcare Team

Understanding your pathology report can be overwhelming due to the technical language and the implications of the findings. It is essential to discuss the results with your healthcare provider, who can explain the terms, answer questions, and discuss how the findings influence your treatment options. Don't hesitate to ask for clarification or further explanation to ensure you are fully informed about your diagnosis and the rationale behind your treatment plan.

Conclusion

The pathology report is a foundational document in the breast cancer diagnosis and treatment process. It provides a detailed snapshot of the cancer's characteristics, guiding the healthcare team in crafting a personalized treatment approach. Patients empowered with knowledge about their pathology report can engage in meaningful conversations with their healthcare providers, contributing to informed decision-making and a sense of control over their treatment journey.

2.4 Exercise: 10 MCQs with Answers at the End

Below are 10 multiple-choice questions designed to test your understanding of the diagnostic journey for breast cancer, including screening methods, biopsy types, and interpreting pathology reports. Find the answers provided at the end to check your knowledge.

1. What is the primary purpose of a mammogram in breast cancer screening?

   A. To remove breast cancer tumors

   B. To diagnose breast cancer with certainty

   C. To detect breast changes or abnormalities early

   D. To determine the best treatment for breast cancer

2. Which biopsy method involves removing a small cylinder of tissue for examination?

   A. Fine Needle Aspiration Biopsy

   B. Core Needle Biopsy

   C. Surgical Biopsy

   D. Stereotactic Biopsy

3. What does a Breast MRI specifically benefit?

   A. Replacing mammograms entirely

   B. Screening women at average risk

   C. Screening women with high breast cancer risk

   D. Confirming breast cancer diagnosis without a biopsy

4. A pathology report stating "positive margins" suggests:

   A. No cancer cells are present at the edge of the biopsy sample.

   B. Cancer cells are found at the edge of the biopsy sample.

   C. The entire tumor has been successfully removed.

   D. There are no cancer cells in the lymph nodes.

5. Tumor grade in a pathology report indicates:

   A. The size of the tumor

   B. How much cancer cells look like healthy cells

   C. The presence of hormone receptors

   D. The effectiveness of the biopsy method used

6. Which is NOT a type of information typically included in a pathology report?

   A. Patient's genetic history

   B. Diagnosis of the breast tissue examined

   C. Hormone receptor status of the tumor

   D. HER2/neu status of the cancer

7. What does ER-positive mean in the context of breast cancer?

   A. The cancer grows in response to excess exercise.

   B. The cancer is resistant to all forms of estrogen.

C. The cancer cells have estrogen receptors and may grow in response to the hormone.

D. The cancer cells are positive for energy recovery.

8. Ultrasound-guided biopsy is most helpful for:

A. Tumors visible on an MRI but not on a mammogram

B. Abnormalities not palpable but visible on ultrasound

C. Determining the HER2 status of a tumor

D. Patients who are allergic to MRI contrast dye

9. HER2/neu status is important because:

A. It determines if a patient is eligible for surgery.

B. It influences the choice of targeted therapies.

C. It indicates the patient's genetic predisposition to cancer.

D. It predicts the speed of tumor growth.

10. Core Needle Biopsy is preferred over Surgical Biopsy for:

A. Providing immediate treatment for breast cancer

B. Removing large tumors entirely

C. Diagnosing cancer without needing surgery

D. Screening women at average risk of breast cancer

Answers:

1. C. To detect breast changes or abnormalities early

2. B. Core Needle Biopsy

3. C. Screening women with high breast cancer risk

4. B. Cancer cells are found at the edge of the biopsy sample.

5. B. How much cancer cells look like healthy cells

6. A. Patient's genetic history

7. C. The cancer cells have estrogen receptors and may grow in response to the hormone.

8. B. Abnormalities not palpable but visible on ultrasound

9. B. It influences the choice of targeted therapies.

10. C. Diagnosing cancer without needing surgery

Chapter 3: Treatment Options

3.1 Surgery: Types and What to Expect

Surgery plays a pivotal role in the treatment of breast cancer, often being the first line of action after a diagnosis. The goal of breast cancer surgery varies from removing as much of the cancer as possible to determining the extent of its spread. This section outlines the main types of breast cancer surgery and what patients might expect before, during, and after the procedure.

Types of Breast Cancer Surgery

- **Lumpectomy (Breast-Conserving Surgery)**: This procedure involves removing the tumor and a small margin of surrounding tissue while preserving most of the breast. It's typically followed by radiation therapy to destroy any remaining cancer cells. Lumpectomy is an option for early-stage breast cancer and allows for breast preservation.

- **Mastectomy**: A mastectomy involves removing one or both breasts, partially (segmental mastectomy) or completely (total mastectomy). The choice between a lumpectomy and mastectomy often depends on the tumor's size, location, and personal preferences. For women at very high risk of developing breast cancer, a prophylactic mastectomy may be considered to reduce this risk.

  - **Simple Mastectomy**: Removal of the entire breast without removing underarm lymph nodes.

  - **Double Mastectomy**: Removal of both breasts, usually as a preventive measure for those at high risk.

  - **Radical Mastectomy**: A more extensive surgery that includes the removal of the breast, underlying chest muscles, and lymph nodes in the armpit. This procedure is rare and usually only recommended when the cancer has spread to the chest muscles.

- **Sentinel Lymph Node Biopsy (SLNB)**: When breast cancer is diagnosed, determining whether it has spread to the lymph nodes is crucial. SLNB involves injecting a radioactive substance or dye near the tumor to identify the first few lymph nodes into which a tumor drains (sentinel nodes). These nodes are then removed and analyzed for cancer cells. If cancer is not found, it's unlikely to have spread to other nodes, possibly eliminating the need for further lymph node removal.

- **Axillary Lymph Node Dissection (ALND)**: If cancer is found in the sentinel nodes, or if there is a high suspicion of lymph node involvement, an ALND may be performed to remove additional lymph nodes from under the arm. This procedure helps define the cancer stage and guide treatment decisions but comes with a higher risk of lymphedema.

What to Expect Before Surgery

Patients will undergo preoperative assessments, including blood tests and, in some cases, imaging tests, to ensure they are fit for surgery. Discussions with the surgical team will cover the surgery's scope, potential risks, and recovery expectations. This is also a time to discuss reconstruction options if a mastectomy is planned.

During Surgery

Surgery length varies depending on the type of procedure. Lumpectomies and sentinel lymph node biopsies are generally shorter and may be done as outpatient procedures, allowing patients to go home the same day. Mastectomies and axillary lymph node dissections are more complex and may require a hospital stay.

After Surgery

Recovery times and experiences vary. Pain, swelling, and tenderness in the treated area are common, and medications are provided for pain management. Physical therapy may be recommended to prevent stiffness and improve range of motion. Patients are monitored for signs of complications, such as infection or lymphedema, and are provided with guidelines for at-home care.

Conclusion

Surgical options for breast cancer treatment are varied and are chosen based on the cancer's characteristics, stage, and patient preferences. Understanding the different types of surgeries and what to expect can help patients feel more prepared and involved in their care decisions. Post-surgical recovery is an important aspect of treatment, with support available to manage physical and emotional recovery.

3.2 Radiation Therapy: Process and Side Effects

Radiation therapy is a common treatment for breast cancer, utilized to destroy cancer cells that may remain after surgery or to reduce the risk of recurrence. This treatment uses high-energy rays or particles to target and kill cancerous cells. Understanding the process and potential side effects of radiation therapy can help patients prepare for what to expect and manage any challenges that may arise during treatment.

The Radiation Therapy Process

- **Consultation and Planning**: Before starting radiation therapy, patients undergo a consultation with a radiation oncologist to discuss the goals and plan the treatment. This is followed by a planning session (simulation), where imaging tests (CT scans) are used to determine the precise location for treatment. Marks may be placed on the skin to guide the placement of radiation beams.

- **Types of Radiation Therapy**:

    - **External Beam Radiation Therapy (EBRT)**: The most common form of radiation therapy for breast cancer, where radiation is directed at the breast from a machine outside the body. Treatments are typically given five days a week for three to six weeks.

    - **Brachytherapy (Internal Radiation)**: Involves placing radioactive material inside the body close to the cancer cells. This is sometimes used after lumpectomy in early-stage breast cancer to deliver radiation directly to the area around the surgery site.

- **Treatment Sessions**: Radiation therapy sessions are quick, often lasting only a few minutes, although preparation time may extend the total visit to about 30 minutes. The process is painless, similar to getting an X-ray.

Side Effects of Radiation Therapy

Side effects from radiation therapy can vary based on the type and dose of radiation, and the area being treated. Common side effects include:

- **Skin Changes**: Redness, blistering, and peeling in the treated area, similar to a sunburn. These typically begin within a few weeks of starting treatment and gradually improve after completing therapy.

- **Fatigue**: Many patients experience fatigue that can persist for weeks to months after treatment concludes.

- **Breast Changes**: The breast may become firmer, swell, or change in size. Some women also report tenderness or a sensation of fullness.

- **Lymphedema**: In cases where the lymph nodes are treated, there's a risk of lymphedema, a condition characterized by swelling due to fluid buildup.

- **Heart and Lung Problems**: For radiation therapy targeting the left side of the chest, there's a slight risk of heart and lung issues, although modern techniques aim to minimize exposure to these organs.

Managing Side Effects

- **Skin Care**: Gentle washing with lukewarm water, using mild soap, and applying recommended creams can help manage skin irritation.

- **Rest**: Prioritizing rest and managing energy levels can help cope with fatigue.

- **Physical Activity**: Light exercise, as tolerated, can improve energy levels and overall well-being.

- **Follow-Up Care**: Regular follow-up appointments are essential for monitoring recovery and managing any long-term side effects.

Conclusion

Radiation therapy is a critical component of breast cancer treatment for many patients, offering a targeted approach to destroying cancer cells. While side effects are common, they are generally manageable with appropriate care and support. Understanding the process and communicating openly with the healthcare team can help patients navigate radiation therapy more comfortably, contributing to a more effective treatment experience.

3.3 Chemotherapy and Biological Therapies

Chemotherapy and biological therapies play a significant role in the treatment of breast cancer, attacking cancer cells with different mechanisms of action. Understanding these treatments, including how they work and their potential side effects, can empower patients to make informed decisions about their care.

Chemotherapy

Chemotherapy uses powerful drugs to kill rapidly dividing cells, a hallmark of cancer cells. However, because chemotherapy can also affect normal cells that divide quickly, it can lead to a range of side effects.

- **How It's Administered**: Chemotherapy can be given intravenously (through a vein) or orally (as pills). The treatment regimen usually consists of cycles, with periods of treatment followed by rest periods to allow the body to recover.

- **Purpose**: It may be used before surgery (neoadjuvant chemotherapy) to shrink a tumor, after surgery (adjuvant chemotherapy) to eliminate any remaining cancer cells, or as the main treatment if cancer has spread beyond the breast and lymph nodes.

Common Side Effects of Chemotherapy

- **Fatigue**

- **Hair Loss**

- **Nausea and Vomiting**

- **Increased Risk of Infection** (due to reduced white blood cell count)

- **Mouth Sores**

- **Changes in Appetite**

- **Changes in Weight**

Management strategies for these side effects include medications to prevent nausea, dietary adjustments, and regular monitoring of blood cell counts to manage infection risk.

Biological (Targeted) Therapies

Biological therapies target specific molecules involved in the growth and spread of cancer cells, sparing most normal cells and potentially resulting in fewer side effects than chemotherapy.

- **Types of Biological Therapies**:

  - **HER2-targeted therapies**: Drugs like trastuzumab (Herceptin) and pertuzumab (Perjeta) target the HER2 protein, which is overexpressed in some breast cancers.

    - **Hormone therapies**: For cancers that are hormone receptor-positive, treatments like tamoxifen or aromatase inhibitors block the body's natural hormones (estrogen and progesterone) from supporting cancer growth.

    - **CDK4/6 inhibitors**: Drugs that target proteins affecting cell division, used in combination with hormone therapy for certain advanced breast cancers.

- **Administration**: Biological therapies can be given intravenously or orally, depending on the specific drug.

Common Side Effects of Biological Therapies

- **Flu-like Symptoms** (fever, chills, weakness)

- **Diarrhea**

- **Skin Rashes**

- **Heart Problems** (especially with some HER2-targeted therapies)

- **Fatigue**

Management of side effects varies with the specific type of biological therapy but may include medications to manage symptoms, lifestyle modifications, and regular monitoring of heart function when necessary.

Conclusion

Chemotherapy and biological therapies are crucial in the multi-faceted approach to treating breast cancer, offering options to attack the disease at different stages and from different angles. While side effects are a significant concern, ongoing advancements in treatment and supportive care continue to improve the quality of life for patients undergoing these therapies. Open communication with healthcare providers about the benefits, risks, and management of side effects is essential for optimizing treatment outcomes and ensuring patient well-being throughout the cancer journey.

3.4 Exercise: 10 MCQs with Answers at the End

Test your understanding of chemotherapy, biological therapies, and their roles in breast cancer treatment with the following multiple-choice questions. Answers are provided at the end for self-assessment.

1. Chemotherapy targets:

   A. Only cancer cells

   B. Rapidly dividing cells

   C. The immune system

   D. Hormone receptors

2. Biological therapies are designed to:

   A. Increase the rate of cell division

   B. Target specific aspects of cancer cells

   C. Suppress the body's natural defense mechanisms

   D. Enhance the effects of chemotherapy by increasing cell sensitivity

3. Neoadjuvant chemotherapy is given:

A. After surgery to prevent recurrence

B. Before radiation therapy to enhance its effects

C. Before surgery to shrink the tumor

D. As the only treatment in metastatic breast cancer

4. Which is NOT a common side effect of chemotherapy?

A. Hair loss

B. Fever

C. High blood pressure

D. Nausea and vomiting

5. HER2-targeted therapies are used for breast cancers that:

A. Lack hormone receptors

B. Are triple-negative

C. Overexpress the HER2 protein

D. Have mutated BRCA genes

6. Hormone therapies are most effective for cancers that are:

A. HER2-positive

B. Hormone receptor-positive

C. Triple-negative

D. Not influenced by hormones

7. Which is a side effect unique to some biological therapies and not typically seen with chemotherapy?

    A. Diarrhea

    B. Skin rashes

    C. Heart problems

    D. Fatigue

8. CDK4/6 inhibitors are used in combination with:

    A. Radiation therapy

    B. Hormone therapy

    C. Chemotherapy

    D. Surgery

9. The purpose of adjuvant chemotherapy is to:

    A. Replace surgical treatment

    B. Shrink tumors before surgery

    C. Eliminate remaining cancer cells after surgery

    D. Act as the sole treatment for advanced cancer

10. A common management strategy for chemotherapy-induced nausea is:

A. Fasting before treatment

B. Physical exercise immediately after treatment

C. Medications to prevent nausea

D. Increasing fluid intake during treatment

Answers:

1. B. Rapidly dividing cells

2. B. Target specific aspects of cancer cells

3. C. Before surgery to shrink the tumor

4. C. High blood pressure

5. C. Overexpress the HER2 protein

6. B. Hormone receptor-positive

7. C. Heart problems

8. B. Hormone therapy

9. C. Eliminate remaining cancer cells after surgery

10. C. Medications to prevent nausea

Chapter 4: Holistic and Complementary Therapies

4.1 Diet and Nutrition

In the comprehensive care of breast cancer, diet and nutrition play pivotal roles, not only in supporting the body through treatment but also in potentially reducing recurrence risks and enhancing overall well-being. This segment explores how dietary choices can impact breast cancer outcomes and offers guidance for adopting a nutrition plan that supports health during and after treatment.

The Role of Diet in Breast Cancer Management

Dietary habits can influence the body's cancer-fighting capabilities, recovery from treatments, and quality of life. While no single food can prevent or cure cancer, a balanced diet rich in certain nutrients can help bolster the immune system, minimize treatment side effects, and reduce the risk of disease progression or recurrence.

Key Dietary Recommendations

- **Plant-Based Foods**: Emphasize a variety of fruits, vegetables, whole grains, and legumes. These foods are high in vitamins, minerals, fiber, and antioxidants, which can help reduce inflammation and improve health.

- **Lean Protein Sources**: Include lean meats, fish, eggs, and plant-based proteins such as beans and lentils. Adequate protein intake is crucial for repairing tissues damaged by cancer treatments and for maintaining muscle mass.

- **Healthy Fats**: Focus on sources of monounsaturated and polyunsaturated fats, such as olive oil, nuts, seeds, and fatty fish like salmon. These fats can support heart health, which is especially important for those undergoing certain types of chemotherapy or hormonal therapies that may impact heart function.

- **Limit Processed and Red Meats**: Studies suggest a link between the consumption of processed and red meats and an increased risk of certain types of cancer. Opting for lean protein sources can be a healthier choice.

- **Reduce Added Sugars and Refined Carbohydrates**: High intake of sugary foods and refined carbs can lead to weight gain and increased cancer risk. Focusing on whole foods can help manage weight and support overall health.

- **Alcohol Consumption**: Alcohol has been linked to an increased risk of breast cancer. Limiting or avoiding alcohol can reduce risk.

- **Stay Hydrated**: Adequate hydration is essential for supporting all bodily functions, including the efficient removal of toxins. Water, herbal teas, and low-sugar beverages can help maintain hydration.

Individualized Nutrition Planning

It's important to recognize that optimal nutrition can vary from person to person, depending on treatment side effects, individual health needs, and specific dietary restrictions. Working with a registered dietitian or a nutritionist who specializes in cancer care can help create a personalized nutrition plan that addresses these unique needs.

Supplements and Breast Cancer

While some may consider dietary supplements to boost nutrient intake, it's essential to consult with a healthcare provider before starting any supplements. Certain vitamins and minerals, especially in high doses, can interact with cancer treatments or have unintended effects on cancer cells.

Conclusion

Integrating a thoughtful approach to diet and nutrition into the breast cancer treatment and recovery plan can play a significant role in enhancing physical health, supporting recovery, and potentially reducing the risk of cancer recurrence. By focusing on a diet rich in whole, nutrient-dense foods, individuals can lay a strong foundation for a healthier future, underscoring the importance of holistic care in the journey through breast cancer.

4.2 Exercise and Physical Well-being

Exercise plays a crucial role in enhancing the quality of life for breast cancer survivors. Regular physical activity can help mitigate the side effects of treatment, reduce the risk of cancer recurrence, and improve overall health outcomes. This section outlines the benefits of exercise for breast cancer survivors and offers guidance on incorporating physical activity into recovery and beyond.

Benefits of Exercise for Breast Cancer Survivors

- **Improved Physical Function**: Exercise can help rebuild strength and flexibility diminished by treatment, aiding in recovery and the return to daily activities.

- **Enhanced Emotional Well-being**: Physical activity has been shown to decrease symptoms of depression and anxiety, improving overall mood and emotional health.

- **Reduced Fatigue**: Although it might seem counterintuitive, regular exercise can combat the persistent tiredness common among cancer survivors.

- **Weight Management**: Keeping a healthy weight is crucial, as excess weight can increase the risk of cancer recurrence and other health issues.

- **Bone Health**: Certain cancer treatments can weaken bones; weight-bearing exercises help maintain bone density and reduce the risk of osteoporosis.

- **Lower Risk of Recurrence and Improved Survival**: Studies have suggested that regular physical activity can reduce the risk of breast cancer recurrence and increase survival rates.

Getting Started with Exercise

Starting an exercise program should be a gradual process, especially after treatment. Here are some guidelines:

- **Consult with Healthcare Providers**: Before beginning any exercise regimen, it's important to get clearance from your healthcare team, particularly if you're dealing with side effects like lymphedema or bone metastasis.

- **Begin Slowly**: Start with low-intensity activities, such as walking or gentle yoga, and gradually increase the intensity and duration as your strength and stamina improve.

- **Incorporate Variety**: A mix of cardiovascular exercises, strength training, flexibility exercises, and balance activities can provide comprehensive health benefits and prevent boredom.

- **Listen to Your Body**: Pay attention to your body's signals and adjust your activities accordingly. Rest when you feel tired, and avoid pushing through pain.

- **Set Realistic Goals**: Establish achievable goals that motivate you without causing undue stress or physical strain.

- **Seek Support**: Joining a cancer survivor exercise group or working with a fitness professional who has experience with cancer survivors can provide encouragement and ensure you're exercising safely.

Safety Considerations

Certain precautions are necessary to ensure safety during exercise, particularly for those with ongoing side effects from treatment:

- **Lymphedema**: If you have or are at risk for lymphedema, wearing a compression garment during exercise may be recommended.

- **Bone Metastasis**: Activities that put excessive stress on bones should be avoided if you have or are at risk for bone metastasis.

- **Neuropathy**: For survivors experiencing neuropathy, balance and strength training can help, but caution is needed to prevent falls.

Conclusion

Incorporating exercise into the recovery process and beyond can offer significant benefits for breast cancer survivors, from improving physical function and emotional well-being to potentially reducing the risk of cancer recurrence. With careful planning and consideration of individual health circumstances, physical activity can be a valuable component of holistic cancer care and survivorship.

4.3 Mind-Body Practices (Yoga, Meditation, etc.)

Mind-body practices such as yoga and meditation have gained recognition for their role in supporting the physical and emotional well-being of breast cancer survivors. These practices focus on the connection between the mind and body, offering tools to manage stress, reduce symptoms of treatment side effects, and enhance overall quality of life. This section explores the benefits of incorporating mind-body practices into the care plan for individuals navigating the journey of breast cancer recovery.

Benefits of Mind-Body Practices

- **Stress Reduction**: Both yoga and meditation are renowned for their ability to lower stress levels. By focusing on the present and fostering a sense of calm, these practices can mitigate the anxiety and stress often associated with cancer diagnosis and treatment.

- **Improved Emotional Well-being**: Engaging in mind-body practices can lead to improvements in mood, reducing feelings of depression and enhancing overall emotional resilience.

- **Enhanced Physical Function**: Yoga, in particular, can improve flexibility, strength, and balance, which may be compromised following cancer treatments such as surgery and chemotherapy.

- **Pain Management**: Regular participation in yoga and meditation has been shown to help reduce pain levels and improve pain tolerance, making these practices beneficial for managing chronic pain and discomfort.

- **Better Sleep**: Many breast cancer survivors experience sleep disturbances. Mind-body practices can improve sleep quality by promoting relaxation and easing the mind.

- **Fatigue Reduction**: By improving sleep, reducing stress, and enhancing physical function, mind-body practices can also help alleviate the persistent fatigue common among cancer survivors.

Incorporating Mind-Body Practices into Your Routine

- **Start with Guided Sessions**: For beginners, starting with guided yoga classes or meditation sessions can provide a foundation in the basics and ensure practices are performed safely.

- **Explore Different Styles**: There are various forms of yoga and meditation. Experimenting with different styles can help you find the ones that best suit your needs and preferences.

- **Create a Regular Practice**: Consistency is key to reaping the benefits. Aim to incorporate these practices into your daily routine, even if only for a few minutes at a time.

- **Adapt Practices to Your Needs**: Mind-body practices are highly adaptable. Modifications can be made to accommodate physical limitations or treatment side effects, ensuring that the practices are both safe and beneficial.

- **Use Resources**: Many resources are available, including online classes, apps, and books, which can guide you in practicing yoga and meditation at home.

Safety Considerations

While mind-body practices are generally safe, certain precautions should be taken, especially during recovery from breast cancer treatment:

- **Consult with Healthcare Providers**: Before starting any new exercise regimen, including yoga and meditation, discuss it with your healthcare team.

- **Listen to Your Body**: Avoid positions or practices that cause pain or discomfort. Use props and modifications as needed to support your body.

- **Hydrate and Nourish**: Ensure you are well-hydrated and have eaten adequately before engaging in physical activities like yoga.

Conclusion

Mind-body practices offer a holistic approach to recovery and well-being for breast cancer survivors, addressing both the physical and emotional aspects of healing. By incorporating practices such as yoga and meditation into your care plan, you can support your journey toward recovery with tools that foster resilience, reduce stress, and enhance quality of life.

4.4 Exercise: 10 MCQs with Answers at the End

Test your knowledge on the integration of holistic and complementary therapies, including diet, exercise, and mind-body practices, in the management and recovery of breast cancer. Find the answers at the end to check your understanding.

1. A diet rich in what type of foods is recommended for breast cancer survivors?

   A. High-fat, low-carbohydrate

   B. Plant-based, high in fruits and vegetables

   C. High in processed meats and sugars

   D. Low-protein, high-dairy

2. Regular physical activity for breast cancer survivors can help:

A. Increase the risk of lymphedema

B. Reduce the risk of cancer recurrence

C. Increase fatigue levels

D. Decrease bone density

3. Yoga can benefit breast cancer survivors by:

A. Increasing stress levels

B. Improving flexibility and strength

C. Worsening sleep quality

D. Reducing heart health

4. Meditation is primarily used to:

A. Enhance physical strength

B. Increase heart rate

C. Reduce stress and anxiety

D. Increase chemotherapy side effects

5. Which of the following is NOT a benefit of a balanced diet in breast cancer management?

A. Reducing the effectiveness of treatments

B. Supporting the immune system

C. Managing weight

D. Reducing inflammation

6. What type of fats are recommended in the diet of a breast cancer survivor?

A. Saturated fats

B. Trans fats

C. Monounsaturated and polyunsaturated fats

D. Hydrogenated fats

7. Incorporating what type of exercise is beneficial for maintaining bone health in breast cancer survivors?

A. Sedentary activities

B. High-impact sports

C. Weight-bearing exercises

D. None; exercise should be avoided

8. Mind-body practices like yoga and meditation can help manage which common side effect of cancer treatment?

A. Hair growth

B. Fatigue

C. Bone metastasis

D. Increased appetite

9. What safety consideration should be taken when a breast cancer survivor starts a yoga practice?

A. Avoid all physical activity

B. Consult with a healthcare provider

C. Only practice in extreme heat conditions

D. Focus solely on cardiovascular exercises

10. Why is hydration important for breast cancer survivors engaging in physical and mind-body practices?

A. It decreases muscle flexibility

B. It increases the risk of lymphedema

C. It supports bodily functions and removes toxins

D. It is not important; focus should be on diet only

Answers:

1. B. Plant-based, high in fruits and vegetables

2. B. Reduce the risk of cancer recurrence

3. B. Improving flexibility and strength

4. C. Reduce stress and anxiety

5. A. Reducing the effectiveness of treatments

6. C. Monounsaturated and polyunsaturated fats

7. C. Weight-bearing exercises

8. B. Fatigue

9. B. Consult with a healthcare provider

10. C. It supports bodily functions and removes toxins

Chapter 5: Living with Breast Cancer

5.1 Managing Side Effects and Symptoms

Living with breast cancer involves navigating a range of side effects and symptoms brought on by the disease itself or as a result of treatments such as surgery, chemotherapy, radiation therapy, and hormone therapy. Effective management of these side effects is crucial for maintaining quality of life and ensuring that patients can continue with their treatment plans. This section offers insights into common side effects and strategies for managing them.

Common Side Effects and Management Strategies

- **Fatigue**: One of the most common side effects experienced by breast cancer patients, fatigue can be managed through regular, gentle exercise; maintaining a healthy diet; and scheduling rest periods throughout the day. Prioritizing activities and practicing good sleep hygiene can also help.

- **Pain**: Pain may result from the cancer itself, surgery, or other treatments. Management strategies include medication, physical therapy, acupuncture, and relaxation techniques such as deep breathing and guided imagery.

- **Lymphedema**: This condition, characterized by swelling in the arm or chest area, can occur after lymph node removal or radiation therapy. Preventive measures include gentle exercises to encourage lymph fluid drainage, wearing a compression garment, and avoiding heavy lifting with the affected arm.

- **Cognitive Changes ("Chemo Brain")**: Symptoms include memory lapses, difficulty concentrating, and troubles with multitasking. Strategies to manage cognitive changes include using tools like planners and lists, engaging in brain-stimulating activities, and regular physical activity.

- **Emotional and Psychological Effects**: Anxiety, depression, and fear of recurrence are common. Support may be found through counseling, support groups, mindfulness practices, and, when necessary, medications to manage symptoms.

- **Changes in Appearance**: Hair loss, weight changes, and surgical scars can affect self-esteem. Wigs, makeup, and prosthesis can help address these concerns, as can support from counseling and support groups.

- **Menopausal Symptoms**: Hormone therapy and chemotherapy can induce menopausal symptoms such as hot flashes, night sweats, and vaginal dryness. Lifestyle adjustments, medications, and non-hormonal therapies can help manage these symptoms.

- **Bone Health**: Some treatments can weaken bones. Calcium and vitamin D supplements, weight-bearing exercises, and medications to protect bone density can be beneficial.

- **Heart Health**: Certain therapies can affect heart health. Regular monitoring, lifestyle changes (diet and exercise), and medications to manage risk factors like high blood pressure and cholesterol can help maintain heart health.

Integrating Side Effect Management into Daily Life

The management of side effects is a dynamic process that requires close communication with the healthcare team. Patients are encouraged to report new symptoms or changes in existing ones promptly. Lifestyle modifications, adherence to prescribed treatments for side effects, and engaging in complementary therapies can significantly enhance well-being.

Additionally, exploring resources such as rehabilitation services, nutritional counseling, and social support networks can provide additional layers of support, helping patients navigate the complexities of living with breast cancer more comfortably.

Conclusion

Managing the side effects and symptoms of breast cancer is an essential component of comprehensive care, enabling patients to lead more comfortable and fulfilling lives despite the challenges of the disease. Through a combination of medical treatments, lifestyle modifications, and support, individuals can find effective strategies to mitigate the impact of side effects on their daily lives.

5.2 Emotional Well-being and Support Networks

The emotional journey of living with breast cancer encompasses a wide range of feelings, from fear and anger to hope and resilience. Emotional well-being is a critical component of overall health, particularly for those navigating the challenges of cancer treatment and survivorship. This section explores the importance of emotional health and the role of support networks in enhancing the quality of life for breast cancer patients.

Understanding the Emotional Impact of Breast Cancer

The diagnosis of breast cancer can trigger a complex mix of emotions, not only for the patient but also for their loved ones. Common feelings include:

- **Anxiety and Fear**: Concerns about the future, treatment outcomes, and the possibility of recurrence are prevalent.

- **Depression**: Feelings of sadness, hopelessness, or loss of interest in activities once enjoyed can occur.

- **Isolation**: Patients may feel alone in their experiences, even when surrounded by supportive friends and family.

- **Guilt**: There may be feelings of guilt about the perceived impact of one's illness on others.

- **Anger**: Frustration and anger about the diagnosis and its consequences are common.

Strategies for Enhancing Emotional Well-being

- **Seek Professional Help**: Counseling or therapy can provide valuable space to process emotions and develop coping strategies. Mental health professionals specializing in oncology can offer tailored support.

- **Join a Support Group**: Connecting with others who have had similar experiences can reduce feelings of isolation and provide practical advice and emotional support.

- **Practice Mindfulness and Relaxation Techniques**: Activities like meditation, yoga, and deep-breathing exercises can help manage stress and anxiety.

- **Stay Active**: Physical activity has been shown to improve mood and reduce symptoms of depression and anxiety.

- **Maintain Social Connections**: Keeping in touch with friends and family, even in small ways, can provide a sense of normalcy and support.

- **Engage in Activities You Enjoy**: Finding time for hobbies and interests can offer a respite from the stress of treatment and recovery.

The Role of Support Networks

Support networks play a crucial role in the emotional well-being of breast cancer patients. These networks can include:

- **Healthcare Team**: Open communication with doctors, nurses, and other healthcare professionals can provide reassurance and clarity about treatment processes and expectations.

- **Family and Friends**: Loved ones can offer emotional support, practical help, and a sense of stability during challenging times.

- **Community Resources**: Local and online support groups, cancer organizations, and community programs can provide additional layers of support, offering opportunities to connect with others and access to various resources.

- **Peer Support**: One-on-one support from someone who has been through a similar experience can be incredibly validating and empowering.

Conclusion

The emotional well-being of breast cancer patients is an integral part of the healing journey. By acknowledging and addressing the complex emotions associated with cancer diagnosis and treatment, and by leveraging the strength of support networks, patients can navigate the path toward recovery with resilience and support. Embracing a comprehensive approach to care that includes emotional, mental, and social health is essential for enhancing the quality of life for those affected by breast cancer.

5.3 Navigating Work and Family Life

For individuals diagnosed with breast cancer, balancing the demands of treatment with work responsibilities and family life presents a unique set of challenges. Adjusting to a new normal while undergoing treatment can strain personal and professional relationships and impact financial stability. This section provides guidance for managing these aspects effectively, ensuring a supportive environment for recovery and maintaining a sense of normalcy.

Balancing Work During Treatment

- **Inform Your Employer**: If comfortable, discuss your diagnosis and treatment plan with your employer. Many organizations offer accommodations, such as flexible hours or the option to work from home, to support employees during this time.

- **Understand Your Rights**: Familiarize yourself with your employment rights under laws such as the Americans with Disabilities Act (ADA) and the Family and Medical Leave Act (FMLA) in the U.S., which can protect your job while you take medical leave.

- **Prioritize Tasks**: Focus on essential responsibilities and consider delegating or postponing less critical tasks. This can help manage workload and reduce stress.

- **Seek Support**: Some workplaces offer support through HR departments, employee assistance programs (EAPs), or support groups for employees dealing with health issues.

Managing Family Life

- **Open Communication**: Share your feelings, fears, and needs with your family. Honest conversations can help manage expectations and foster a supportive home environment.

- **Accept Help**: Allow friends and family to assist with daily tasks such as childcare, household chores, or meal preparation. Accepting help can alleviate some of the burdens and provide loved ones with practical ways to support you.

- **Protect Time for Self-Care**: Prioritize activities that promote your well-being, such as exercise, hobbies, or relaxation techniques. Self-care is crucial for maintaining emotional resilience.

- **Consider Counseling**: Family counseling or support groups can be beneficial for addressing the emotional impact of cancer on relationships and helping families navigate the challenges together.

Financial Considerations

- **Review Insurance Coverage**: Understand your health insurance benefits and any out-of-pocket costs associated with your treatment. This can help prevent unexpected financial strains.

- **Explore Financial Assistance**: Many organizations offer financial aid, grants, or resources to help cover the costs of cancer treatment and related expenses.

- **Budgeting**: Adjusting your budget to accommodate medical expenses and potentially reduced income is essential. Financial advisors or counselors can offer guidance tailored to your situation.

Creating a Supportive Work and Family Environment

- **Educate Colleagues and Family Members**: Sharing information about breast cancer and its treatments can help others understand what you're going through and how they can offer support.

- **Set Boundaries**: Communicate your limits regarding work and social commitments. Setting boundaries can help manage energy levels and reduce the risk of burnout.

- **Plan for the Future**: Work with your healthcare team to anticipate changes in your condition or treatment needs. This can help you make informed decisions about work and family responsibilities.

Conclusion

Navigating work and family life while managing breast cancer is a balancing act that requires communication, support, and flexibility. By seeking accommodations, understanding your rights, and prioritizing your health and well-being, you can create a supportive environment that accommodates your needs during treatment and recovery. Remember, it's okay to ask for help and make adjustments as needed to maintain your quality of life and focus on healing.

5.4 Exercise: 10 MCQs with Answers at the End

Test your understanding of the complexities of living with breast cancer, focusing on managing side effects, supporting emotional well-being, navigating work and family life, and understanding financial implications. Check your answers at the end to gauge your comprehension.

1. What is a common strategy to manage treatment-related fatigue?

   A. Increase caffeine intake

   B. Regular, gentle exercise

   C. Avoid all physical activity

   D. Sleep less to promote nighttime rest

2. Effective pain management for breast cancer patients may include:

   A. Ignoring the pain until it resolves on its own

   B. Only using prescription opioids

   C. Utilizing a combination of medication and acupuncture

   D. Increasing alcohol consumption

3. Lymphedema, a potential side effect of treatment, can be managed by:

   A. Wearing tight clothing to compress the area

   B. Engaging in high-intensity weight lifting

   C. Using a compression garment and practicing gentle exercises

   D. Completely avoiding movement of the affected limb

4. A beneficial practice for managing "chemo brain" includes:

   A. Avoiding mentally stimulating activities

   B. Using planners and lists for organization

   C. Increasing screen time before bed

   D. Consuming alcohol to relax the brain

5. When navigating work during treatment, it's important to:

A. Keep your diagnosis and treatment a secret from your employer

B. Understand your rights under employment and health laws

C. Refuse any offered accommodations to prove resilience

D. Immediately quit your job upon diagnosis

6. Open communication with family about your breast cancer journey helps to:

A. Eliminate all stress within the household

B. Manage expectations and foster a supportive environment

C. Ensure family members will not feel any emotional impact

D. Shift all responsibilities back to the patient

7. Financial assistance for managing the costs associated with breast cancer treatment can be sought through:

A. Only personal loans

B. Health insurance and financial aid organizations

C. Avoiding all medical treatments to save money

D. Selling personal belongings as the only option

8. Emotional well-being can be enhanced by:

    A. Isolating oneself from friends and family

    B. Ignoring feelings of anxiety and depression

    C. Seeking professional help and joining support groups

    D. Avoiding any form of physical activity

9. Managing work-life balance during breast cancer treatment involves:

    A. Overworking to distract from the diagnosis

    B. Setting clear boundaries and seeking flexible work arrangements

    C. Keeping work and treatment schedules completely separate

    D. Not informing your healthcare team about your work

10. A key aspect of self-care for breast cancer survivors is:

    A. Neglecting personal interests and hobbies

    B. Prioritizing activities that promote well-being

    C. Staying up late to complete work or household chores

    D. Limiting intake of water and nutritious foods

Answers:

1. B. Regular, gentle exercise

2. C. Utilizing a combination of medication and acupuncture

3. C. Using a compression garment and practicing gentle exercises

4. B. Using planners and lists for organization

5. B. Understand your rights under employment and health laws

6. B. Manage expectations and foster a supportive environment

7. B. Health insurance and financial aid organizations

8. C. Seeking professional help and joining support groups

9. B. Setting clear boundaries and seeking flexible work arrangements

10. B. Prioritizing activities that promote well-being

Chapter 6: Breast Cancer in Special Populations

6.1 Young Women with Breast Cancer

Breast cancer in young women, typically defined as those diagnosed under the age of 40, presents unique challenges and considerations. This population faces distinct issues related to treatment, fertility, genetic risk, and emotional well-being. Understanding these aspects is crucial for providing appropriate support and care.

Unique Challenges Faced by Young Women

- **Biological Aggressiveness**: Breast cancer in young women often tends to be more aggressive and to be diagnosed at a later stage than in older women. The cancers may be more likely to be triple-negative or HER2-positive.

- **Fertility Concerns**: Treatments such as chemotherapy and hormonal therapy can impact fertility. Young women may need to consider fertility preservation options, like egg or embryo freezing, before starting treatment.

- **Genetic and Family Risk**: Younger women diagnosed with breast cancer have a higher likelihood of having a genetic predisposition to the disease, such as BRCA1 or BRCA2 mutations. This can have implications for both their treatment plan and their family members.

- **Psychosocial Impact**: The diagnosis can profoundly affect young women's lives, impacting their careers, relationships, and plans for having children. They may also feel isolated from peers who are not facing similar health issues.

Treatment Considerations

- **Personalized Treatment Plans**: Treatment decisions should consider the tumor's characteristics, the woman's age, and her personal preferences, including thoughts on fertility and concerns about side effects.

- **Fertility Preservation**: Discussions about fertility should be part of the treatment planning process. Referral to a fertility specialist before starting treatment can provide information on preservation options.

- **Genetic Testing and Counseling**: Given the higher risk of a genetic component, genetic testing and counseling are recommended for young women with breast cancer. This can inform treatment decisions and implications for family members.

Supporting Emotional Well-being

- **Peer Support**: Connecting with other young women who have experienced breast cancer can provide valuable support and reduce feelings of isolation.

- **Counseling and Mental Health Services**: Professional support can help navigate the emotional and psychological challenges of a breast cancer diagnosis and treatment.

- **Comprehensive Care Teams**: Including specialists in oncology, fertility, genetics, and psychology can provide a holistic approach to care, addressing the wide range of needs specific to young women with breast cancer.

Conclusion

Breast cancer in young women requires a tailored approach that addresses the biological, reproductive, and emotional aspects unique to this population. Early and aggressive treatment, combined with supportive care that includes fertility preservation, genetic counseling, and psychosocial support, is essential for managing the disease and supporting young women through their breast cancer journey. Establishing a supportive network and utilizing resources designed for young breast cancer survivors can enhance quality of life and outcomes.

6.2 Male Breast Cancer: Overlooked but Important

Although breast cancer is most commonly associated with women, it's crucial to acknowledge that men can also be diagnosed with the disease. Male breast cancer is rare, accounting for less than 1% of all breast cancer cases, but it carries significant health implications. The rarity of breast cancer in men can lead to late diagnosis and treatment, underscoring the need for awareness and understanding.

Understanding Male Breast Cancer

- **Risk Factors**: Key risk factors for male breast cancer include age (most common in men over 60), family history of breast cancer, genetic mutations (such as BRCA1 and BRCA2), radiation exposure, and elevated levels of estrogen.

- **Symptoms**: Similar to women, men should be vigilant for changes in breast tissue, such as lumps, skin dimpling or puckering, nipple retraction, redness, and discharge.

- **Diagnosis and Treatment**: Diagnostic tests for male breast cancer are similar to those used for women, including mammograms, ultrasounds, and biopsies. Treatment options also parallel those for female breast cancer, encompassing surgery, radiation therapy, chemotherapy, and hormonal therapy, depending on the cancer's characteristics.

Challenges and Considerations

- **Awareness and Stigma**: A lack of awareness and societal stigma around male breast cancer can delay men from seeking medical advice for symptoms, leading to diagnoses at more advanced stages.

- **Emotional Impact**: Men with breast cancer may face unique psychological challenges, including feelings of isolation due to the rarity of their condition. Support groups and counseling services tailored to men can provide essential emotional support.

- **Genetic Counseling**: Men diagnosed with breast cancer should consider genetic testing and counseling, as they may carry gene mutations that increase their risk for other cancers and have implications for family members.

Support and Resources

- **Education**: Increasing education and awareness about male breast cancer is crucial for early detection and treatment. Men should be informed about the signs of breast cancer and encouraged to report changes to their healthcare providers.

- **Support Networks**: Access to support networks, including those specifically for men with breast cancer, can help address the feeling of isolation and provide a platform for sharing experiences and advice.

- **Comprehensive Care**: A multidisciplinary approach to treatment, involving oncologists, genetic counselors, and mental health professionals, can ensure that men receive tailored care that addresses all aspects of their well-being.

Conclusion

Male breast cancer, while rare, is an important public health issue that requires increased awareness and understanding. By promoting education on the signs and risk factors, and by providing supportive resources tailored to men, healthcare providers can enhance the detection, treatment, and support for men affected by breast cancer. Addressing the unique challenges faced by men with breast cancer can lead to better outcomes and improve the quality of life for those diagnosed with this overlooked condition.

6.3 Geriatric Oncology: Breast Cancer in the Elderly

Breast cancer in elderly patients, typically defined as those aged 65 and older, presents unique challenges in diagnosis, treatment, and management. The growing population of older adults increases the importance of understanding how to best care for this group, taking into account the complexities of aging and coexisting health conditions.

Challenges in Treating Elderly Breast Cancer Patients

- **Coexisting Conditions**: Older patients often have other health issues, such as heart disease, diabetes, or osteoporosis, which can complicate cancer treatment and affect prognosis.

- **Functional Status**: Assessing an elderly patient's functional status, including their ability to perform daily activities and live independently, is crucial in treatment planning.

- **Treatment Tolerance**: Elderly patients may have a reduced capacity to tolerate standard cancer treatments due to decreased organ function and reserve.

- **Underrepresentation in Clinical Trials**: Older adults are often underrepresented in clinical trials, leading to a gap in evidence-based guidelines for this population.

Considerations for Treatment

- **Personalized Treatment Plans**: Treatment decisions should be individualized, taking into account the patient's overall health, life expectancy, and preferences. The potential benefits of treatment must be weighed against the risks and potential impact on quality of life.

- **Comprehensive Geriatric Assessment (CGA)**: A CGA can help evaluate an elderly patient's medical, functional, and psychosocial status, guiding treatment choices and support needs.

- **Minimally Invasive Options**: Whenever possible, less aggressive and minimally invasive treatments may be considered to reduce side effects and recovery time.

- **Management of Side Effects**: Elderly patients require careful monitoring for treatment-related side effects, with prompt management to prevent complications.

Supporting Quality of Life

- **Multidisciplinary Approach**: A team that includes oncologists, geriatricians, nurses, social workers, and physical therapists can address the diverse needs of elderly breast cancer patients.

- **Social Support**: Ensuring strong social support networks, including family, friends, and community resources, is vital for the emotional well-being of elderly patients.

- **Palliative Care**: Incorporating palliative care early in the treatment process can help manage symptoms and improve quality of life, regardless of the prognosis.

Ethical Considerations

- **Autonomy and Decision Making**: Respecting the autonomy and treatment preferences of elderly patients is essential. Discussions about goals of care, advanced directives, and palliative care options should be part of the care process.

- **Avoiding Ageism**: Treatment decisions should not be based solely on age. Elderly patients with breast cancer deserve the same thoughtful, individualized approach to care as younger patients.

Conclusion

Breast cancer treatment in the elderly requires a tailored approach that balances the benefits and risks of treatment against the backdrop of aging and coexisting health conditions. By adopting a comprehensive, multidisciplinary strategy that emphasizes quality of life and respects patient preferences, healthcare providers can offer effective, compassionate care to elderly breast cancer patients. This approach ensures that age alone does not dictate the scope or nature of treatment, allowing for dignified and personalized care.

6.4 Exercise: 10 MCQs with Answers at the End

This exercise tests your knowledge on the unique considerations and challenges of managing breast cancer in special populations, including young women, men, and the elderly. Check your answers at the end to see how well you understand these important topics.

1. Breast cancer in young women often tends to be:

    A. Less aggressive than in older women

    B. Diagnosed at an earlier stage

    C. More likely to be hormone receptor-positive

    D. More aggressive and diagnosed at a later stage

2. A key consideration for young women undergoing breast cancer treatment is:

    A. Fertility preservation

    B. Immediate enrollment in support groups

    C. Avoiding all forms of physical activity

    D. Starting treatment without genetic testing

3. Male breast cancer is:

    A. More common than in females

    B. Typically less aggressive than in females

    C. Often diagnosed at a later stage due to lack of awareness

    D. Unaffected by genetic factors

4. In the treatment of elderly breast cancer patients, it's important to:

A. Apply the same treatment protocols as for younger patients

B. Consider the patient's overall health and coexisting conditions

C. Exclude them from all forms of chemotherapy

D. Focus solely on palliative care

5. Genetic testing and counseling in young women with breast cancer can:

A. Guarantee a cure

B. Increase the risk of developing other cancers

C. Inform treatment decisions and implications for family members

D. Be skipped if the patient is under 30

6. The primary reason elderly breast cancer patients may have a reduced capacity to tolerate standard treatments is:

A. Overrepresentation in clinical trials

B. Increased organ function and reserve

C. Decreased organ function and reserve

D. Lack of symptoms

7. One way to support the emotional well-being of men with breast cancer is to:

A. Isolate them from other cancer patients

B. Provide access to male-specific support groups

C. Discourage any form of emotional expression

D. Ignore any signs of psychological distress

8. A Comprehensive Geriatric Assessment (CGA) in elderly breast cancer patients is used to:

A. Determine the patient's favorite color

B. Evaluate the patient's medical, functional, and psychosocial status

C. Convince the patient to refuse treatment

D. Assess the patient's ability to drive

9. Fertility concerns for young women with breast cancer are addressed through:

A. Immediate surgery

B. Fertility preservation options before starting treatment

C. Advising patients to ignore fertility issues

D. Limiting treatment options to surgery only

10. The importance of multidisciplinary care in treating elderly breast cancer patients is to:

A. Simplify treatment by using a single therapy

B. Address diverse needs beyond just the cancer treatment

C. Increase the use of aggressive treatments

D. Focus exclusively on physical health without considering emotional well-being

Answers:

1. D. More aggressive and diagnosed at a later stage

2. A. Fertility preservation

3. C. Often diagnosed at a later stage due to lack of awareness

4. B. Consider the patient's overall health and coexisting conditions

5. C. Inform treatment decisions and implications for family members

6. C. Decreased organ function and reserve

7. B. Provide access to male-specific support groups

8. B. Evaluate the patient's medical, functional, and psychosocial status

9. B. Fertility preservation options before starting treatment

10. B. Address diverse needs beyond just the cancer treatment

Chapter 7: Advances in Breast Cancer Research

7.1 Genetic Research and BRCA Mutations

Genetic research has significantly advanced our understanding of breast cancer, particularly in identifying BRCA1 and BRCA2 gene mutations, which increase the risk of developing breast and ovarian cancers. This section delves into the impact of genetic research on breast cancer, focusing on BRCA mutations, their implications for risk assessment, prevention strategies, and personalized treatment approaches.

Understanding BRCA Mutations

BRCA1 and BRCA2 genes help repair damaged DNA, playing a crucial role in maintaining the genetic material's integrity. Mutations in these genes can lead to DNA repair errors, accumulating mutations that can initiate cancer development. Individuals with inherited mutations in BRCA1 or BRCA2 have a significantly increased risk of developing breast and ovarian cancers compared to the general population.

Implications of BRCA Mutations

- **Risk Assessment**: Genetic testing for BRCA mutations can identify individuals at high risk for breast and ovarian cancers, allowing for proactive surveillance and risk-reduction strategies.

- **Preventive Measures**: Options for individuals with BRCA mutations include increased surveillance (such as more frequent mammograms and MRI screenings), chemoprevention (medications like tamoxifen), and prophylactic surgeries (preventive removal of breasts and/or ovaries).

- **Family Planning**: Knowing one's BRCA status can also inform family planning decisions, as these mutations can be passed to offspring.

Advances in Treatment

- **Targeted Therapies**: BRCA mutations have paved the way for targeted therapies, such as PARP inhibitors, which specifically target cancer cells with defective DNA repair mechanisms, sparing healthy cells and reducing side effects.

- **Personalized Medicine**: Genetic information about BRCA mutations helps tailor treatment plans to individual patients, optimizing outcomes by selecting therapies most likely to be effective based on a tumor's genetic profile.

The Future of Genetic Research in Breast Cancer

Ongoing research aims to uncover additional genetic factors contributing to breast cancer risk and to develop new targeted therapies. Efforts are also focused on understanding the mechanisms behind BRCA mutations' resistance to certain treatments and on identifying markers that predict treatment response.

Ethical and Social Considerations

The ability to test for BRCA mutations raises ethical and social issues, including concerns about privacy, genetic discrimination, and the psychological impact of knowing one's genetic risk. Counseling before and after genetic testing is crucial to help individuals make informed decisions and cope with the results.

Conclusion

Genetic research, particularly on BRCA mutations, has revolutionized the approach to breast cancer risk assessment, prevention, and treatment. As our understanding of the genetic underpinnings of breast cancer deepens, the potential for more effective, personalized therapies grows. However, navigating the complexities of genetic information requires careful consideration of the ethical, psychological, and social implications.

7.2 The Future of Immunotherapy

Immunotherapy represents a groundbreaking shift in the battle against breast cancer, harnessing the body's immune system to recognize and attack cancer cells. This emerging field has shown promising results, offering new hope for treatments that are both effective and have fewer side effects compared to traditional methods. The future of immunotherapy in breast cancer care is rapidly evolving, with research focusing on developing more targeted, personalized approaches.

Understanding Immunotherapy

Immunotherapy works by enhancing the innate powers of the immune system, helping it to identify and combat cancerous cells. Several types of immunotherapy are being explored in breast cancer, including:

- **Checkpoint Inhibitors**: These drugs block proteins that prevent the immune system from attacking cancer cells, allowing T-cells to more effectively destroy these cells.

- **Monoclonal Antibodies**: Designed to target specific antigens on cancer cells, these antibodies can block cancer growth signals, mark cancer cells for destruction, or deliver toxic substances directly to cancer cells.

- **Cancer Vaccines**: Aimed at preventing cancer recurrence, these vaccines stimulate the immune system to attack cancer cells by recognizing specific cancer-associated antigens.

- **Adoptive Cell Therapy**: This involves enhancing a patient's own immune cells (like T-cells) outside the body before reintroducing them to target and kill cancer cells.

Challenges and Opportunities

While immunotherapy offers a promising new avenue for breast cancer treatment, several challenges remain:

- **Identifying Responders**: Currently, only a subset of breast cancer patients responds to immunotherapy. Research is focused on identifying biomarkers that predict which patients will benefit most.

- **Combination Therapies**: Combining immunotherapy with other treatments, such as chemotherapy, targeted therapy, or radiation, may enhance effectiveness and overcome resistance mechanisms.

- **Managing Side Effects**: Although generally less toxic than chemotherapy, immunotherapies can cause immune-related adverse effects. Developing strategies to manage these side effects is crucial.

The Future of Immunotherapy in Breast Cancer

The future of immunotherapy in breast cancer treatment is focused on:

-   **Personalized Medicine**: Tailoring immunotherapies to individual patient profiles and tumor characteristics to maximize effectiveness and minimize side effects.

- **New Targets and Technologies**: Discovering new immune targets and developing innovative delivery methods to enhance the precision and efficacy of immunotherapies.

- **Combination Strategies**: Exploring synergistic combinations of immunotherapies and other cancer treatments to improve outcomes for a broader range of patients.

- **Preventive Vaccines**: Researching vaccines that could prevent breast cancer in high-risk individuals or prevent recurrence in those who have been treated.

Conclusion

Immunotherapy holds significant promise for transforming breast cancer treatment, moving towards more personalized, less toxic, and more effective therapies. As research advances, the hope is that immunotherapy will become a cornerstone of breast cancer care, offering improved outcomes and quality of life for patients. The ongoing exploration of the immune system's role in cancer will likely uncover new avenues for treatment, prevention, and possibly even cures in the future.

7.3 Personalized Medicine and Targeted Therapies

Personalized medicine, also known as precision medicine, represents a paradigm shift in the treatment of breast cancer, moving away from a one-size-fits-all approach to a more tailored strategy. This approach leverages detailed information about an individual's genetic makeup and the specific characteristics of their tumor to customize treatment plans. Targeted therapies play a crucial role in this personalized approach, offering the potential for more effective treatments with fewer side effects.

Principles of Personalized Medicine

- **Genetic Profiling**: By analyzing the genetic mutations within a cancer cell, doctors can identify specific drivers of an individual's cancer. This information guides the selection of targeted therapies that will be most effective against those drivers.

- **Biomarker Testing**: Biomarkers are molecular signs of a specific process or condition, and their presence can help predict how well a certain cancer will respond to a treatment. Tests for biomarkers like hormone receptors (ER, PR) and HER2 are standard in breast cancer care, determining eligibility for hormonal therapies and HER2-targeted treatments.

- **Risk Stratification**: Genetic and molecular information can also help stratify patients by risk, identifying those who might benefit from more aggressive treatment versus those who can avoid unnecessary side effects from treatments unlikely to provide benefit.

Advancements in Targeted Therapies

Targeted therapies focus on specific cellular pathways or genetic markers involved in cancer growth and spread. Recent advancements include:

- **HER2-targeted Therapies**: For cancers that overexpress the HER2 protein, drugs such as trastuzumab, pertuzumab, and ado-trastuzumab emtansine have significantly improved outcomes.

- **Hormone Receptor-targeted Therapies**: For ER-positive cancers, treatments targeting the estrogen receptor, such as tamoxifen and aromatase inhibitors, are effective in preventing recurrence.

- **PARP Inhibitors**: For patients with BRCA mutations, PARP inhibitors like olaparib and talazoparib can specifically target cancer cells' DNA repair pathways, leading to cell death.

- **CDK4/6 Inhibitors**: Drugs like palbociclib, ribociclib, and abemaciclib target proteins involved in cell division, used in combination with hormonal therapy for advanced ER-positive breast cancer.

Challenges and Future Directions

While personalized medicine and targeted therapies offer hope for more effective breast cancer treatment, challenges remain:

- **Cost and Accessibility**: The high cost of genetic testing and targeted therapies may limit access for some patients.

- **Resistance**: Cancer cells can develop resistance to targeted therapies, necessitating ongoing research to find new targets and treatment combinations.

- **Complexity of Cancer**: The genetic complexity of tumors and their ability to evolve over time means that a single targeted therapy may not be effective for all patients, highlighting the need for combination treatments and continuous monitoring.

Conclusion

Personalized medicine and targeted therapies are at the forefront of transforming breast cancer treatment, offering a more scientific and tailored approach to care. By focusing on the genetic and molecular characteristics of each patient's cancer, these approaches aim to optimize treatment effectiveness, minimize side effects, and improve overall outcomes. As research continues to evolve, the hope is that increasingly sophisticated treatments will become available, making breast cancer a more manageable and even curable disease for many patients.

7.4 Exercise: 10 MCQs with Answers at the End

Test your knowledge on the latest advances in breast cancer research, including genetic research, immunotherapy, personalized medicine, and targeted therapies. Evaluate your understanding and check the answers provided at the end.

1. What do BRCA1 and BRCA2 genes help to repair?

   A. Bone fractures

   B. Muscle tissue

   C. Damaged DNA

   D. Blood vessels

2. Personalized medicine in breast cancer treatment primarily relies on:

   A. The patient's age and gender

   B. Generic treatment protocols

   C. Genetic profiling of the tumor

   D. The number of previous treatments

3. Which type of therapy targets the HER2 protein in breast cancer cells?

A. Hormone therapy

B. Chemotherapy

C. HER2-targeted therapy

D. Radiation therapy

4. PARP inhibitors are especially effective for patients with mutations in which genes?

A. APOE

B. BRCA1 and BRCA2

C. CDK4/6

D. HER2

5. Immunotherapy works by:

A. Directly attacking cancer cells with chemicals

B. Enhancing the body's immune system to fight cancer

C. Blocking blood supply to the tumor

D. Repairing damaged DNA in cancer cells

6. The main advantage of targeted therapies over traditional chemotherapy is:

A. They are less expensive

B. They have no side effects

C. They are effective for all cancer types

D. They can specifically target cancer cells, reducing harm to normal cells

7. Which of the following is a challenge in the use of personalized medicine?

A. It simplifies treatment decisions

B. It is universally accessible and affordable

C. Resistance to targeted therapies may develop

D. There are too few options for targeted therapies

8. A major focus of breast cancer research is:

A. Decreasing the use of surgery

B. Developing vaccines to prevent breast cancer

C. Eliminating the need for radiation therapy

D. Using chemotherapy as the sole treatment option

9. Biomarkers in breast cancer are used to:

   A. Determine the patient's blood type

   B. Predict how well a cancer will respond to a treatment

   C. Measure the physical strength of a patient

   D. Assess the patient's psychological readiness for treatment

10. The role of CDK4/6 inhibitors in breast cancer treatment is to:

   A. Stimulate the immune system

   B. Target proteins involved in cell division

   C. Reduce the side effects of chemotherapy

   D. Increase the effectiveness of radiation therapy

Answers:

1. C. Damaged DNA

2. C. Genetic profiling of the tumor

3. C. HER2-targeted therapy

4. B. BRCA1 and BRCA2

5. B. Enhancing the body's immune system to fight cancer

6. D. They can specifically target cancer cells, reducing harm to normal cells

7. C. Resistance to targeted therapies may develop

8. B. Developing vaccines to prevent breast cancer

9. B. Predict how well a cancer will respond to a treatment

10. B. Target proteins involved in cell division

Chapter 8: Prevention Strategies

8.1 Lifestyle Changes and Risk Reduction

While not all cases of breast cancer can be prevented, evidence suggests that lifestyle choices can significantly impact the risk of developing the disease. This section explores practical lifestyle adjustments and behaviors that can contribute to reducing breast cancer risk, emphasizing the importance of a proactive approach to health and wellness.

Maintaining a Healthy Weight

Obesity and being overweight have been linked to an increased risk of developing breast cancer, particularly after menopause. A healthy weight can be maintained through:

- **Balanced Diet**: Focusing on a diet rich in fruits, vegetables, whole grains, and lean proteins while limiting processed foods, red meat, and high-fat dairy products.

- **Regular Physical Activity**: Engaging in at least 150 minutes of moderate aerobic activity or 75 minutes of vigorous activity each week, alongside muscle-strengthening exercises.

Physical Activity

Regular exercise not only aids in maintaining a healthy weight but also offers independent protective effects against breast cancer. The benefits include:

- **Hormone Regulation**: Physical activity can help regulate hormones, including estrogen and insulin, which can influence breast cancer risk.

- **Immune Function**: Exercise may enhance the body's immune response, helping to protect against cancer formation.

Limiting Alcohol Intake

Alcohol consumption is a known risk factor for breast cancer. Limiting alcohol to no more than one drink per day—or avoiding it altogether—can reduce risk.

Smoking Cessation

Smoking is associated with a higher risk of many cancers, including breast cancer. Quitting smoking at any age can lower the risk of breast cancer, in addition to providing numerous other health benefits.

Dietary Considerations

Certain dietary patterns may be associated with a reduced risk of breast cancer:

- **Plant-based Diets**: Diets high in fruits, vegetables, and whole grains and low in processed foods and red meat.

- **Antioxidant-rich Foods**: Foods high in antioxidants, such as berries, nuts, and green leafy vegetables, may help protect against cell damage.

Breastfeeding

Breastfeeding for a total of one year or more cumulatively for all children can lower the risk of breast cancer for mothers.

Chemoprevention

For women at high risk of breast cancer, medications such as tamoxifen or raloxifene may be recommended to reduce risk. Decisions about chemoprevention should be made in consultation with a healthcare provider.

Conclusion

Adopting a healthy lifestyle can play a significant role in reducing the risk of breast cancer. While genetic and environmental factors also influence risk, lifestyle changes offer a proactive way to potentially lower that risk and enhance overall health. Awareness and education about these strategies are key components of prevention efforts, empowering individuals to make informed choices about their health and well-being.

8.2 Screening and Early Detection Strategies

Screening and early detection are pivotal in the fight against breast cancer. Early-stage breast cancers are more likely to be treated successfully, highlighting the importance of regular screening to identify cancers before they cause symptoms. This section outlines the recommended screening strategies and their role in reducing breast cancer mortality.

Mammography

The most widely recommended screening method for breast cancer is mammography, an X-ray exam of the breast. Mammography can detect tumors that are too small to feel and can show if a tumor is likely benign or cancerous.

- **Recommendations**: Guidelines vary, but most health organizations recommend that women start regular mammograms at age 40 to 50 and continue annually or biennially until at least age 74. Women with a higher risk of breast cancer may need to start screening earlier and more frequently.

Breast Magnetic Resonance Imaging (MRI)

Breast MRI is a more sensitive screening tool than mammography and is recommended for women at high risk for breast cancer. This includes women with a known BRCA1 or BRCA2 gene mutation, a family history of breast cancer, or other risk factors.

- **Use with Mammography**: For high-risk women, breast MRI is often used in addition to, not instead of, mammography, because each method can catch cancers the other might miss.

Clinical Breast Exams and Self-Exams

While mammography and MRI play central roles in breast cancer screening, clinical breast exams (performed by healthcare professionals) and breast self-exams can also be part of a comprehensive screening strategy.

- **Clinical Breast Exams**: These may be recommended every 1 to 3 years for women in their 20s and 30s and annually for women 40 and older.

- **Breast Self-Exams**: Women are encouraged to be familiar with their breasts so they can notice any changes and report them to their healthcare provider. However, self-exams should not replace mammograms or clinical exams.

Risk-Based Screening

Recognizing that breast cancer risk varies from person to person, some experts advocate for risk-based screening strategies that tailor screening recommendations based on an individual's specific risk factors.

- **Genetic Counseling and Testing**: For women with family histories suggestive of a genetic risk for breast cancer, genetic counseling followed by testing for mutations in genes like BRCA1 and BRCA2 can inform personalized screening plans.

Emerging Screening Technologies

Research is ongoing to improve breast cancer screening and early detection. This includes developing new imaging technologies, blood tests for cancer markers, and genetic tests that could offer more precise risk assessments.

Conclusion

Effective screening and early detection strategies are critical for reducing breast cancer mortality. Adherence to recommended screening schedules, combined with awareness of personal risk factors, can significantly impact early detection rates. As research advances, screening guidelines may continue to evolve, further improving outcomes for women worldwide.

8.3 Vaccination and Future Preventative Measures

The concept of using vaccines to prevent breast cancer is an area of active research and represents a promising frontier in the fight against this disease. While no vaccine currently exists to prevent breast cancer in the general population, developments in this field could drastically change the landscape of cancer prevention. Additionally, exploring other future preventative measures offers hope for reducing the incidence of breast cancer.

Breast Cancer Vaccines

- **Therapeutic Vaccines**: Current research primarily focuses on therapeutic vaccines, which aim to prevent the recurrence of breast cancer in individuals who have already been diagnosed with the disease. These vaccines are designed to train the immune system to recognize and attack cancer cells.

- **Prophylactic Vaccines**: Prophylactic (preventative) vaccines, which would aim to prevent breast cancer from developing in the first place, are also under investigation. These vaccines would target specific proteins or antigens associated with breast cancer cells.

Mechanisms and Targets

- **Targeting Antigens**: Breast cancer vaccines under development aim to target specific antigens found on the surface of cancer cells. By stimulating the body's immune response against these antigens, the vaccine could potentially prevent the cancer from developing or recurring.

- **HER2 Protein**: Some vaccines target the HER2 protein, which is overexpressed in a subset of breast cancers. Early-phase clinical trials have shown promise in preventing recurrence in patients with HER2-positive breast cancer.

Challenges in Vaccine Development

- **Complexity of Breast Cancer**: The heterogeneity of breast cancer, meaning the wide variety of types and molecular characteristics, complicates the development of a universal vaccine.

- **Immune Tolerance**: The body's natural tolerance to its own tissues can make it challenging to develop a vaccine that effectively targets tumor cells without harming normal cells.

Future Preventative Measures

Beyond vaccines, ongoing research into breast cancer prevention includes:

- **Genetic and Molecular Profiling**: Identifying individuals at high risk for breast cancer through genetic and molecular profiling could lead to targeted prevention strategies.

- **Lifestyle Interventions**: Research continues to explore the role of diet, exercise, and other lifestyle factors in breast cancer prevention, aiming to provide evidence-based recommendations.

- **Chemoprevention**: The use of drugs to reduce cancer risk in high-risk individuals is another area of focus. Further studies aim to identify effective agents with minimal side effects.

Conclusion

The development of vaccines and other preventative measures against breast cancer represents a promising area of research with the potential to significantly impact public health. While challenges remain, the ongoing exploration of therapeutic and prophylactic vaccines, along with advancements in understanding the genetic and lifestyle factors contributing to breast cancer risk, holds promise for future prevention strategies. As science progresses, the hope is that one day it will be possible to prevent breast cancer before it ever begins, reducing the global burden of this disease.

8.4 Exercise: 10 MCQs with Answers at the End

Evaluate your knowledge of breast cancer prevention strategies, including lifestyle changes, screening, and future preventative measures. Check your answers at the end to see how well you understand these critical aspects of reducing breast cancer risk.

1. Regular physical activity can reduce breast cancer risk by:

   A. Increasing estrogen levels

   B. Decreasing immune function

   C. Regulating hormones and enhancing immune function

   D. Directly reducing tumor size

2. The primary screening method for breast cancer is:

   A. Clinical breast exam

   B. Breast self-exam

   C. Mammography

   D. MRI

3. A risk factor for breast cancer that individuals can modify is:

   A. Age

   B. Genetic mutations

   C. Alcohol consumption

   D. Family history

4. Breast cancer vaccines currently under research are primarily:

   A. Prophylactic, to prevent initial occurrence in healthy individuals

   B. Therapeutic, to prevent recurrence in those previously diagnosed

   C. Available for general public use

   D. Used to replace chemotherapy

5. Maintaining a healthy weight impacts breast cancer risk by:

   A. Increasing hormone levels associated with risk

   B. Having no impact on breast cancer risk

   C. Potentially reducing the risk, especially after menopause

   D. Solely improving self-esteem

6. Limiting alcohol intake is recommended because alcohol:

   A. Has no impact on cancer risk

B. Can directly cause breast tissue mutations

C. Is associated with an increased risk of breast cancer

D. Decreases the effectiveness of breast cancer treatments

7. Breastfeeding has been shown to:

    A. Increase breast cancer risk

    B. Have no effect on breast cancer risk

    C. Reduce the mother's risk of breast cancer

    D. Only benefit the child's health

8. High-risk women might undergo enhanced screening with:

    A. Additional clinical breast exams only

    B. Breast MRI in addition to mammography

    C. Breast self-exams exclusively

    D. Avoidance of all screening methods

9. A lifestyle factor NOT associated with breast cancer risk is:

    A. High-fat diet

    B. Physical inactivity

    C. Hair dye use

    D. Smoking

10. Future breast cancer prevention strategies include:

A. Discouraging genetic testing for high-risk individuals

B. Developing vaccines to prevent recurrence and possibly initial occurrence

C. Eliminating all current treatment options in favor of lifestyle changes

D. Recommending alcohol intake to manage stress

Answers:

1. C. Regulating hormones and enhancing immune function

2. C. Mammography

3. C. Alcohol consumption

4. B. Therapeutic, to prevent recurrence in those previously diagnosed

5. C. Potentially reducing the risk, especially after menopause

6. C. Is associated with an increased risk of breast cancer

7. C. Reduce the mother's risk of breast cancer

8. B. Breast MRI in addition to mammography

9. C. Hair dye use

10. B. Developing vaccines to prevent recurrence and possibly initial occurrence

Chapter 9: The Role of Technology in Diagnosis and Treatment

9.1 Imaging Technologies: MRI, Mammography, and Ultrasound

Advancements in imaging technologies have significantly improved the diagnosis and treatment of breast cancer, offering more precise detection, characterization, and monitoring of tumors. This section explores the critical roles of MRI, mammography, and ultrasound in breast cancer care.

Mammography

Mammography remains the cornerstone of breast cancer screening. By providing detailed X-ray images of the breast, mammography can detect tumors that are too small to be felt and identify suspicious areas that may require further investigation.

- **Digital Mammography**: Offers clearer images than traditional film mammography, especially beneficial for women under 50 and those with dense breast tissue.

- **3D Mammography (Tomosynthesis)**: Creates a three-dimensional picture of the breast, improving the detection of breast cancer and reducing the need for follow-up imaging.

Magnetic Resonance Imaging (MRI)

Breast MRI uses magnetic fields and radio waves to produce detailed images of the breast. It is particularly useful in specific situations:

- **High-Risk Screening**: Recommended for women at high risk of breast cancer, such as those with a known BRCA mutation, a strong family history, or other genetic predispositions.

- **Assessing the Extent of Cancer**: Helps determine the size of the cancer, detect additional tumors in the breast, and assess involvement of chest wall structures or lymph nodes.

- **Evaluating Treatment Response**: Used to monitor how well neoadjuvant (pre-surgery) therapy is working.

Ultrasound

Breast ultrasound utilizes sound waves to create images of the breast tissue. It serves several important functions in breast cancer diagnosis and management:

- **Differentiating Solid Masses from Fluid-filled Cysts**: Ultrasound can help determine if a breast lump is solid (suggesting a tumor) or filled with fluid (a cyst).

- **Guiding Needle Biopsies**: Ultrasound guidance can be used during a biopsy to ensure accurate sampling of the suspicious area.

- **Supplementing Mammography**: Especially useful in women with dense breast tissue, where mammography alone may not be sufficient.

The Integration of Imaging Technologies

The use of these imaging technologies is often complementary, providing a comprehensive view of the breast that aids in accurate diagnosis and effective treatment planning. The choice of imaging technique depends on individual factors such as age, breast density, risk factors, and the specific clinical scenario.

Future Directions

Emerging technologies and ongoing research aim to further enhance the accuracy, efficiency, and accessibility of breast imaging. Innovations such as artificial intelligence and machine learning algorithms are being explored to improve image analysis and interpretation, potentially leading to earlier detection and personalized treatment strategies.

Conclusion

Imaging technologies like MRI, mammography, and ultrasound play indispensable roles in the early detection, diagnosis, and management of breast cancer. As technology advances, the potential for even more precise and personalized breast cancer care becomes increasingly attainable, promising improved outcomes for patients worldwide.

9.2 AI and Machine Learning in Breast Cancer

Artificial Intelligence (AI) and machine learning are at the forefront of revolutionizing breast cancer diagnosis, treatment, and research. These technologies harness vast amounts of data to uncover patterns, predict outcomes, and personalize patient care in ways previously unimaginable. This section explores how AI and machine learning are being applied in the fight against breast cancer.

Enhancing Diagnostic Accuracy

- **Image Analysis**: AI algorithms can analyze mammograms, MRIs, and ultrasound images with high precision, identifying subtle signs of breast cancer that may be missed by the human eye. This capability not only improves diagnostic accuracy but also reduces false positives and negatives, potentially leading to earlier detection and treatment.

- **Pathology Slide Interpretation**: Machine learning tools can evaluate pathology slides from biopsies or surgeries, distinguishing between benign and malignant cells and identifying tumor characteristics critical for staging and treatment planning.

Predicting Treatment Responses and Outcomes

- **Personalized Treatment Plans**: AI models can predict how individual patients will respond to various treatments based on their unique genetic makeup, tumor characteristics, and other clinical data. This information helps clinicians tailor treatment strategies to maximize effectiveness and minimize side effects.

- **Prognostic Models**: Machine learning algorithms can analyze clinical data to predict patient outcomes, such as the risk of recurrence or survival rates. These models assist in making informed decisions about the intensity of treatment needed and in monitoring patients more closely who are at higher risk.

Drug Discovery and Development

- **Identifying New Targets**: AI can sift through vast biological datasets to identify potential new drug targets for breast cancer. This accelerates the pace of discovery and the development of targeted therapies.

- **Optimizing Clinical Trials**: Machine learning can help design clinical trials by selecting patients most likely to benefit from a particular therapy, thereby increasing the trial's efficiency and the likelihood of successful outcomes.

Improving Patient Care and Support

- **Symptom Management**: AI-driven applications can monitor patient-reported symptoms in real-time, enabling timely interventions to manage side effects and improve quality of life.

- **Support Systems**: Chatbots and virtual assistants, powered by AI, provide 24/7 support and information to patients, helping them navigate the complexities of treatment and care.

Challenges and Considerations

While AI and machine learning offer immense promise, there are challenges to their implementation, including data privacy concerns, the need for large, diverse datasets to train algorithms, and ensuring these technologies complement rather than replace the human element in healthcare.

Conclusion

AI and machine learning are transforming the landscape of breast cancer care, offering innovative solutions for early detection, personalized treatment, and patient support. As these technologies continue to evolve, they hold the potential to significantly improve outcomes and quality of life for breast cancer patients, heralding a new era in oncology.

9.3 Telemedicine and Remote Healthcare

Telemedicine and remote healthcare have emerged as essential components of breast cancer care, especially highlighted by the COVID-19 pandemic's challenges. These digital health services enable patients to receive timely consultations, follow-up care, and support from the comfort of their homes, minimizing the need for physical hospital visits and thereby reducing exposure to potential infections. This section explores the role of telemedicine in breast cancer management and its implications for future care.

Benefits of Telemedicine in Breast Cancer Care

- **Access to Specialists**: Telemedicine allows patients, especially those in remote or underserved areas, to consult with breast cancer specialists and multidisciplinary teams they might not otherwise have access to.

- **Convenience and Efficiency**: Virtual appointments can often be more convenient and less time-consuming for patients, eliminating travel time and costs, and reducing the stress associated with hospital visits.

- **Continuous Monitoring**: Wearable devices and mobile health apps can facilitate continuous monitoring of patients' health status, treatment side effects, and medication adherence, allowing for timely interventions when necessary.

- **Psychological Support**: Telemedicine provides avenues for psychological counseling and support group meetings, helping patients cope with the emotional challenges of breast cancer diagnosis and treatment.

Integrating Telemedicine into Breast Cancer Care

- **Virtual Consultations**: Initial consultations, genetic counseling, and follow-up appointments can be effectively conducted via video conferencing, ensuring continuous patient engagement and care.

- **Digital Imaging Reviews**: Radiologists and oncologists can review and discuss imaging results with patients remotely, making diagnostic processes more efficient.

- **Remote Symptom Management**: Patients can report symptoms and side effects through telehealth platforms, receiving prompt advice and adjustments to their treatment plans without needing in-person visits.

- **Education and Rehabilitation**: Telemedicine platforms offer opportunities for patient education on breast cancer, treatment options, and self-care practices, as well as virtual rehabilitation programs to support physical recovery.

Challenges and Future Directions

While telemedicine has proven invaluable in providing care during the pandemic and beyond, challenges remain:

- **Equity and Access**: Ensuring all patients have access to the necessary technology and internet connectivity is crucial for equitable care.

- **Regulatory and Reimbursement Issues**: Adapting regulatory frameworks and insurance policies to support telehealth services is necessary for their sustained integration into healthcare systems.

- **Data Security and Privacy**: Safeguarding patient data and ensuring privacy in digital communications are paramount.

- **Blending Traditional and Digital Care**: Finding the optimal balance between in-person and remote care to maintain the quality and personal touch of healthcare services.

Conclusion

Telemedicine and remote healthcare have significantly enhanced the continuum of care for breast cancer patients, offering flexible, accessible, and efficient care options. As technology advances and healthcare systems adapt, telemedicine is poised to play an increasingly central role in breast cancer management, complementing traditional care models and driving innovations in patient-centered care.

9.4 Exercise: 10 MCQs with Answers at the End

Test your understanding of the role of technology in the diagnosis and treatment of breast cancer, including imaging technologies, AI and machine learning, telemedicine, and more. Review your knowledge and verify your answers provided at the end.

1. Which imaging technology is recommended for women at high risk for breast cancer?

   A. X-ray

   B. MRI

   C. CT scan

   D. PET scan

2. AI and machine learning can enhance breast cancer care by:

   A. Replacing the need for doctors

   B. Providing emotional support to patients

   C. Improving diagnostic accuracy and predicting treatment responses

   D. Performing surgeries

3. The primary benefit of telemedicine in breast cancer care includes:

   A. Physical examinations over the internet

   B. Increased need for hospital visits

   C. Access to specialists and convenience for patients

   D. Elimination of in-person support groups

4. 3D mammography is also known as:

   A. Digital mammography

   B. Tomosynthesis

   C. Ultrasound

   D. MRI

5. Which is NOT a direct application of AI in breast cancer treatment?

   A. Analyzing mammograms for early detection

   B. Predicting patient outcomes based on genetic data

   C. Automatically scheduling patient appointments

   D. Identifying new drug targets

6. Breast MRI is particularly useful for:

   A. All women as a standard screening tool

   B. Women with dense breast tissue and high risk of breast cancer

   C. Replacing mammography completely

   D. Patients without any risk factors

7. Telemedicine can facilitate all except:

   A. Virtual consultations

   B. Remote symptom management

   C. Physical biopsy procedures

   D. Psychological counseling

8. A significant challenge in the implementation of AI in healthcare is:

   A. Too few data available for analysis

   B. Data privacy and security concerns

   C. AI's inability to learn over time

   D. Complete replacement of human judgment

9. Wearable devices in breast cancer care primarily help in:

   A. Administering chemotherapy remotely

   B. Continuous monitoring of health status

C. Performing surgical procedures

D. Directly destroying cancer cells

10. The integration of telemedicine into breast cancer care has been significantly accelerated by:

A. The invention of the internet

B. Advances in surgical techniques

C. The COVID-19 pandemic

D. The development of new chemotherapy drugs

Answers:

1. B. MRI

2. C. Improving diagnostic accuracy and predicting treatment responses

3. C. Access to specialists and convenience for patients

4. B. Tomosynthesis

5. C. Automatically scheduling patient appointments

6. B. Women with dense breast tissue and high risk of breast cancer

7. C. Physical biopsy procedures

8. B. Data privacy and security concerns

9. B. Continuous monitoring of health status

10. C. The COVID-19 pandemic

Chapter 10: Survivorship and Life After Cancer

10.1 Long-term Side Effects of Treatment

Breast cancer survivorship is a journey that extends well beyond the completion of treatment. While the end of active treatment is a significant milestone, survivors often face long-term side effects that can impact their quality of life. This section explores common long-term side effects of breast cancer treatments and strategies for managing them.

Common Long-term Side Effects

- **Lymphedema**: A condition characterized by swelling, usually in the arm or hand, that can occur after lymph node removal or radiation therapy. Management includes physical therapy, compression garments, and careful skin care to prevent infection.

- **Cognitive Changes ("Chemo Brain")**: Difficulties with memory, concentration, and multitasking may persist for months or even years after chemotherapy. Cognitive rehabilitation programs and strategies like routine structuring and mental exercises can help.

- **Menopausal Symptoms**: Treatments that affect hormonal balance, such as chemotherapy and hormone therapy, can induce menopause or worsen its symptoms, including hot flashes, night sweats, and vaginal dryness. Lifestyle changes, non-hormonal medications, and, in some cases, hormone replacement therapy (under strict medical supervision) can alleviate these symptoms.

- **Bone Health**: Chemotherapy and hormone therapies can lead to decreased bone density and increased risk of osteoporosis. Calcium and vitamin D supplements, weight-bearing exercises, and medications to strengthen bones are recommended.

- **Cardiovascular Health**: Some breast cancer treatments can increase the risk of heart problems later in life. Regular cardiovascular screenings and adopting heart-healthy habits (like a balanced diet, regular exercise, and smoking cessation) are crucial.

- **Emotional and Psychological Effects**: Anxiety, depression, and fear of recurrence are common among survivors. Support groups, counseling, and, in some cases, medications can provide significant relief.

Strategies for Managing Long-term Side Effects

- **Regular Follow-up Care**: Ongoing appointments with healthcare providers are essential for monitoring and managing long-term side effects. These visits are opportunities to discuss any new or worsening symptoms.

- **Healthy Lifestyle**: A balanced diet, regular physical activity, and adequate sleep contribute to overall well-being and can mitigate some side effects.

- **Rehabilitation Services**: Physical, occupational, and speech therapy can address specific issues related to physical function, mobility, and cognitive changes.

- **Emotional Support**: Connecting with others through support groups or counseling services can help survivors navigate the emotional challenges of life after cancer.

Conclusion

Survivorship and life after breast cancer involve adjusting to a new normal, where managing long-term side effects is a significant part of the journey. By understanding these potential challenges and implementing strategies to address them, survivors can improve their quality of life and focus on their recovery and well-being. Collaboration with a healthcare team, support from loved ones, and access to survivorship resources are key components of successful long-term care.

10.2 Surveillance and Follow-up Care

Surveillance and follow-up care are integral components of the post-treatment phase for breast cancer survivors. This ongoing care aims to monitor for cancer recurrence, manage long-term side effects of treatment, and address the comprehensive health needs of survivors. Effective follow-up care is tailored to each survivor's unique medical history and treatment experience, ensuring that any new health issues are identified and managed promptly.

Components of Surveillance and Follow-up Care

- **Regular Medical Check-ups**: These include physical exams and discussions about health and any symptoms that might suggest a recurrence of cancer or the emergence of new health issues.

- **Mammograms**: Annual mammograms are typically recommended for detecting breast cancer recurrence or new breast cancers. The frequency and type of imaging may vary based on individual risk factors and treatment history.

- **Monitoring for Recurrence**: In addition to mammography, survivors may undergo other tests and scans as deemed necessary by their healthcare team, based on specific symptoms or concerns.

- **Managing Long-term Side Effects**: Follow-up visits are opportunities to assess and address ongoing side effects from treatment, such as lymphedema, bone density loss, and menopausal symptoms.

- **Psychosocial Support**: Emotional and psychological support remains crucial after treatment ends. Counseling, support groups, and survivorship programs can provide valuable spaces for survivors to share experiences and receive support.

- **Lifestyle and Wellness Counseling**: Advice on nutrition, physical activity, smoking cessation, and other lifestyle factors can help survivors improve their overall health and reduce the risk of cancer recurrence.

Personalized Follow-up Care Plans

Follow-up care should be personalized, taking into account:

- **Type of Breast Cancer and Treatment Received**: The nature of the initial cancer and the treatments a survivor has undergone influence the follow-up care plan.

- **Risk of Recurrence**: Higher-risk individuals may require more frequent monitoring.

- **Individual Health Concerns**: Other health conditions can affect the approach to follow-up care.

Importance of Self-Advocacy

Survivors are encouraged to be proactive in their follow-up care:

- **Communication**: Openly discussing symptoms, concerns, and lifestyle changes with healthcare providers can enhance the effectiveness of follow-up care.

- **Education**: Understanding their health situation enables survivors to make informed decisions about their care and lifestyle choices.

- **Self-Monitoring**: Being aware of changes in their bodies and reporting these changes promptly can help in early detection of recurrence or new health issues.

Conclusion

Surveillance and follow-up care are critical for maintaining the health and well-being of breast cancer survivors. Through regular medical check-ups, monitoring for recurrence, managing long-term side effects, and providing psychosocial support, healthcare providers can help survivors navigate life after breast cancer. Personalized care plans and self-advocacy play vital roles in ensuring that the specific needs of each survivor are met, fostering a proactive approach to health maintenance and quality of life improvements.

10.3 Rebuilding Your Life and Moving Forward

After completing breast cancer treatment, many survivors face the challenge of rebuilding their lives and finding a new normal. This phase involves not only physical recovery but also emotional healing, redefining personal relationships, and adjusting to changes in professional life. Moving forward requires resilience, support, and proactive planning to embrace life beyond cancer.

Physical Recovery and Wellness

- **Exercise and Physical Activity**: Gradually resuming or starting a new exercise routine can help rebuild strength, improve mood, and enhance overall health. Tailor activities to your energy levels and interests.

- **Nutrition**: Adopting a balanced diet rich in fruits, vegetables, whole grains, and lean proteins can support recovery and contribute to long-term health.

- **Rest and Sleep**: Prioritize adequate rest and establish a regular sleep routine to help your body heal and recover energy.

Emotional and Psychological Healing

- **Acknowledge Your Feelings**: It's normal to experience a range of emotions after treatment. Allow yourself to process these feelings, whether through journaling, art, or talking with a trusted friend or therapist.

- **Seek Support**: Joining support groups or connecting with other survivors can provide valuable perspectives and encouragement. Consider professional counseling to navigate emotional challenges and coping strategies.

Redefining Relationships

- **Communication**: Openly discuss your needs, fears, and expectations with loved ones. Cancer can change relationships, and clear communication is essential for understanding and support.

- **Intimacy and Sexuality**: Physical changes and emotional stress can affect intimacy. Be patient with yourself and communicate with your partner about your feelings and concerns. Professional guidance may help in addressing these issues.

Professional Life

- **Gradual Return to Work**: If returning to work, consider a phased approach or flexible scheduling initially. Communicate with your employer about your needs and any adjustments required to support your return.

- **Career Goals**: Reflect on your professional goals and aspirations. Cancer can shift priorities, leading some to pursue new directions in their careers or personal lives.

Long-term Health Management

- **Regular Medical Follow-up**: Continue with scheduled medical appointments and screenings to monitor for any signs of recurrence and manage ongoing health issues.

- **Preventive Care**: Stay informed about preventive measures, including vaccinations and screenings for other health conditions.

Embracing Life Beyond Cancer

- **Find Meaning**: Many survivors find new meaning in their experiences by volunteering, advocating for cancer awareness, or exploring new hobbies and interests.

- **Set Goals**: Setting short-term and long-term goals can provide direction and motivation as you rebuild your life.

Conclusion

Rebuilding life after breast cancer is a deeply personal journey that encompasses physical, emotional, and social dimensions. Embracing change, seeking support, and focusing on what brings joy and fulfillment can guide survivors as they navigate this phase. Moving forward is not just about surviving but thriving, finding strength in the experience, and living life to the fullest with resilience and hope.

10.4 Exercise: 10 MCQs with Answers at the End

Test your understanding of the journey of survivorship and life after breast cancer, covering aspects like managing long-term side effects, follow-up care, rebuilding life, and more. Check your answers at the end to assess your knowledge.

1. Which is an effective strategy for managing lymphedema?

   A. Ignoring swelling and continuing normal activities

   B. Wearing a compression garment and engaging in gentle exercises

C. Applying heat directly to the swollen area

D. Increasing salt intake to promote fluid retention

2. Cognitive changes post-treatment can be managed through:

A. Avoiding mentally stimulating activities

B. Cognitive rehabilitation and mental exercises

C. Increasing caffeine consumption

D. Permanent cognitive decline acceptance

3. A key component of emotional healing after breast cancer treatment is:

A. Isolating oneself to avoid overburdening others

B. Acknowledging feelings and seeking support

C. Avoiding talking about the cancer experience

D. Focusing solely on physical recovery

4. The role of regular medical follow-up in survivorship care includes:

A. Only addressing new cancer occurrences

B. Monitoring for recurrence and managing long-term side effects

C. Discontinuing all medications to test the body's natural healing

D. Focusing exclusively on emotional well-being

5. For breast cancer survivors, maintaining a balanced diet is recommended to:

A. Immediately reverse treatment side effects

B. Support physical recovery and contribute to long-term health

C. Guarantee prevention of cancer recurrence

D. Replace the need for follow-up care

6. Gradual return to work for survivors is advised to:

A. Quickly return to pre-cancer performance levels

B. Allow adjustment to work while managing energy levels

C. Prove to employers the illness has no lasting effects

D. Avoid discussing any workplace accommodations

7. In rebuilding relationships post-cancer, important factors include:

A. Ceasing all previous relationships for new ones

B. Open communication about needs and expectations

C. Assuming loved ones understand all needs without discussion

D. Limiting social interactions to avoid stress

8. Regular physical activity for survivors is recommended to:

   A. Only focus on weight loss

   B. Rebuild strength, improve mood, and enhance health

   C. Avoid any form of exercise due to risk of injury

   D. Solely as a method for social interaction

9. Post-treatment, professional counseling is utilized to:

   A. Discuss only physical health concerns

   B. Navigate emotional challenges and develop coping strategies

   C. Avoid dealing with any cancer-related issues

   D. Replace the need for medical follow-up

10. Setting goals post-treatment helps survivors:

   A. Ignore any past experiences with cancer

   B. Provide direction and motivation as they rebuild their lives

   C. Focus only on cancer-related objectives

   D. Immediately return to their pre-cancer lifestyle

Answers:

1. B. Wearing a compression garment and engaging in gentle exercises

2. B. Cognitive rehabilitation and mental exercises

3. B. Acknowledging feelings and seeking support

4. B. Monitoring for recurrence and managing long-term side effects

5. B. Support physical recovery and contribute to long-term health

6. B. Allow adjustment to work while managing energy levels

7. B. Open communication about needs and expectations

8. B. Rebuild strength, improve mood, and enhance health

9. B. Navigate emotional challenges and develop coping strategies

10. B. Provide direction and motivation as they rebuild their lives

Chapter 11: Legal and Ethical Considerations

11.1 Patient Rights and Privacy

Navigating breast cancer involves not just medical treatment but also understanding and advocating for one's rights as a patient, especially regarding privacy and confidentiality. Legal frameworks, such as the Health Insurance Portability and Accountability Act (HIPAA) in the United States, are designed to protect patients' medical information while ensuring they receive respectful, informed, and confidential care.

Understanding Patient Rights

Patients diagnosed with breast cancer have specific rights, including:

- **Right to Informed Consent**: Before undergoing any procedure or treatment, patients have the right to be fully informed about their options, the risks and benefits, and any potential side effects or complications.

- **Right to Privacy and Confidentiality**: Patients' health information is protected, and details about their diagnosis, treatment, and prognosis cannot be disclosed without their consent.

- **Right to Access Medical Records**: Patients can request and obtain copies of their medical records, allowing them to review their treatment history and make informed decisions about their care.

- **Right to Second Opinion**: Seeking a second opinion is a patient's right, ensuring they have explored all possible options and are comfortable with their treatment plan.

- **Right to Non-Discrimination**: Patients should receive care without discrimination based on age, gender, race, sexual orientation, or any other characteristic.

Navigating Privacy and Confidentiality

- **HIPAA and Similar Regulations**: Laws like HIPAA provide guidelines on how healthcare providers and insurers can use and share patients' health information, emphasizing the importance of protecting patient privacy.

- **Employment Protections**: Legal protections also extend to the workplace, where employers are required to maintain confidentiality regarding an employee's medical condition and provide reasonable accommodations under laws like the Americans with Disabilities Act (ADA).

Ethical Considerations in Patient Care

- **Respect for Autonomy**: Healthcare providers must respect patients' autonomy, allowing them to make their own informed decisions about treatment and care.

- **Beneficence and Non-Maleficence**: The principles of beneficence (acting in the patient's best interest) and non-maleficence (avoiding harm) guide ethical patient care, ensuring that treatment plans are developed with the patient's well-being in mind.

Advocating for Patient Rights

- **Education and Awareness**: Understanding their rights empowers patients to advocate for themselves, ensuring they receive the highest standard of care.

- **Support Resources**: Various organizations and resources are available to help patients navigate the legal and ethical aspects of breast cancer care, offering guidance on patient rights, privacy issues, and advocacy.

Conclusion

Legal and ethical considerations play a crucial role in breast cancer care, with patient rights and privacy at the forefront of ensuring respectful, informed, and confidential treatment. By understanding their rights and advocating for themselves, breast cancer patients can navigate their care with confidence, supported by the legal protections and ethical standards that govern healthcare practice.

11.2 Ethical Issues in Genetic Testing

Genetic testing for breast cancer, particularly for BRCA1 and BRCA2 gene mutations, has become an invaluable tool in assessing risk and guiding treatment decisions. However, the introduction of genetic testing into clinical practice has also raised several ethical issues that need careful consideration.

Privacy and Confidentiality

- **Risk of Discrimination**: There's concern about genetic information being used to discriminate against individuals in employment, insurance, and other areas of life. Laws like the Genetic Information Nondiscrimination Act (GINA) in the U.S. are designed to prevent such discrimination, but concerns persist globally.

- **Family Implications**: The results of genetic testing can have implications for family members, raising questions about whether and how this information should be shared. This involves balancing the individual's right to privacy with the potential benefits of informing relatives about their risk.

Informed Consent

- **Understanding Risks and Benefits**: Obtaining informed consent for genetic testing involves ensuring that patients fully understand the potential risks and benefits, including the emotional and psychological impact of knowing one's genetic risk for cancer.

- **Pressure and Coercion**: Patients must not feel coerced into undergoing genetic testing by healthcare providers or family members. The decision should be voluntary and well-informed.

Psychological Impact

- **Anxiety and Distress**: The knowledge gained from genetic testing can cause significant anxiety and distress, not only for those who test positive for a mutation but also for individuals who receive inconclusive or negative results yet still have a family history of breast cancer.

- **Support and Counseling**: Genetic counseling before and after testing is crucial to help individuals understand the implications of their test results and cope with the emotional and psychological impact.

Equity and Access

- **Accessibility**: There's concern that genetic testing and the benefits it brings may not be equally accessible to all populations, particularly those from underrepresented or economically disadvantaged backgrounds.

- **Cultural Sensitivity**: Different cultures may have varying perceptions of risk, disease, and family obligations, affecting decisions about genetic testing and the sharing of genetic information.

Reproductive Decisions

- **Impact on Reproductive Choices**: For individuals with a high genetic risk of breast cancer, the knowledge gained from genetic testing can influence decisions about reproduction, including options like preimplantation genetic diagnosis (PGD) to prevent passing the mutation to offspring.

Conclusion

The ethical landscape of genetic testing for breast cancer is complex, encompassing issues of privacy, informed consent, psychological impact, equity, and more. Navigating these challenges requires a multidisciplinary approach, involving genetic counselors, ethicists, healthcare providers, and legal experts, to ensure that patients receive compassionate, ethical care that respects their autonomy and rights.

11.3 Navigating Insurance and Financial Assistance

The financial impact of breast cancer treatment can be significant, making insurance coverage and financial assistance crucial components of care. Navigating these aspects requires understanding the coverage options, rights under various health laws, and available resources for financial support. This section provides an overview of navigating insurance issues and seeking financial assistance for breast cancer patients.

Understanding Insurance Coverage

- **Health Insurance Plans**: Review your health insurance policy to understand what treatments, medications, and services are covered. This includes chemotherapy, radiation therapy, surgery, reconstructive surgery, and potentially genetic testing.

- **Pre-authorization**: Some treatments may require pre-authorization from your insurance provider. Understanding this process is essential to ensure coverage.

- **Appealing Denials**: If your insurance denies coverage for a necessary treatment, you have the right to appeal the decision. Familiarize yourself with your insurer's appeal process.

Rights Under Health Laws

- **The Affordable Care Act (ACA)**: In the United States, the ACA provides protections for patients, including prohibiting denial of coverage based on pre-existing conditions and allowing young adults to stay on their parent's insurance until age 26.

- **The Women's Health and Cancer Rights Act (WHCRA)**: Requires health plans that cover mastectomies to also cover reconstructive surgery and certain other post-mastectomy benefits.

- **Medicare and Medicaid**: These government programs offer health coverage for eligible elderly, disabled individuals, and those with low income. Understanding your eligibility and benefits can provide additional support.

Financial Assistance Programs

- **Patient Assistance Programs**: Many pharmaceutical companies offer patient assistance programs for medications at reduced cost or for free to eligible individuals.

- **Non-profit Organizations and Charities**: Numerous organizations offer grants, assistance with travel and lodging expenses, and other financial support for breast cancer patients.

- **Crowdfunding**: Online platforms can be used to raise funds for medical expenses, allowing the community to support patients through donations.

Tips for Navigating Financial Challenges

- **Seek Help from a Financial Navigator**: Many hospitals and cancer centers have financial counselors or navigators who can help you understand your insurance coverage, out-of-pocket costs, and eligibility for assistance programs.

- **Keep Detailed Records**: Maintain records of all treatments, expenses, and communications with your insurance company. This documentation is vital for appeals and for tracking deductible and out-of-pocket maximums.

- **Explore All Options**: Don't hesitate to reach out to social workers, patient advocacy groups, and local community resources for assistance and advice on managing financial aspects of cancer care.

Conclusion

Navigating insurance and financial assistance is a critical but complex part of managing breast cancer care. By understanding your insurance coverage, knowing your rights, and utilizing available resources, you can mitigate some of the financial burdens of treatment. Proactive communication, thorough documentation, and seeking support from financial counselors and advocacy organizations can empower patients and their families to focus more on recovery and less on financial stress.

11.4 Exercise: 10 MCQs with Answers at the End

Test your knowledge on the legal and ethical considerations in breast cancer care, including patient rights and privacy, genetic testing, navigating insurance, and financial assistance. Check your answers at the end to assess your understanding.

1. The Genetic Information Nondiscrimination Act (GINA) protects individuals from discrimination based on:

A. Income level

B. Genetic information

C. Marital status

D. Employment history

2. Informed consent for medical procedures ensures patients are:

A. Automatically enrolled in the most expensive treatment

B. Fully aware of the risks and benefits before agreeing to treatment

C. Not allowed to ask questions about their treatment options

D. Required to undergo genetic testing

3. A key ethical issue in genetic testing for breast cancer is:

   A. The color of the testing kit

   B. Sharing results with family members who may also be at risk

   C. Mandatory participation in clinical trials

   D. Immediate eligibility for all treatment options

4. Health Insurance Portability and Accountability Act (HIPAA) focuses on:

   A. Speeding up insurance claims

   B. Protecting patient health information and privacy

   C. Increasing healthcare costs

   D. Limiting patient access to medical records

5. An appeal can be filed if an insurance company:

   A. Offers too many coverage options

   B. Denies coverage for a necessary treatment

   C. Charges a copay for office visits

   D. Provides excellent customer service

6. Financial assistance for breast cancer patients may include help from:

   A. Only government programs

   B. Pharmaceutical patient assistance programs and non-profit organizations

   C. Credit card companies

   D. Luxury brands

7. One of the patient rights under the Affordable Care Act (ACA) is:

   A. Coverage denial based on pre-existing conditions

   B. Unlimited insurance premiums

   C. Staying on a parent's insurance plan until age 26

   D. Automatic enrollment in experimental treatments

8. Emotional support for navigating legal and ethical considerations can come from:

   A. Watching television

   B. Engaging with support groups and counseling

   C. Ignoring the issues

   D. Only speaking with lawyers

9. The Women's Health and Cancer Rights Act (WHCRA) ensures coverage for:

   A. All forms of cancer treatment, regardless of cost

   B. Reconstructive surgery after mastectomy

   C. Unlimited spa treatments

   D. Personal chefs and nutritionists

10. One challenge in implementing AI in healthcare is:

   A. The complete accuracy of AI predictions

   B. AI's inability to process large data sets

   C. Data privacy and security concerns

   D. AI replacing all human healthcare providers

Answers:

1. B. Genetic information

2. B. Fully aware of the risks and benefits before agreeing to treatment

3. B. Sharing results with family members who may also be at risk

4. B. Protecting patient health information and privacy

5. B. Denies coverage for a necessary treatment

6. B. Pharmaceutical patient assistance programs and non-profit organizations

7. C. Staying on a parent's insurance plan until age 26

8. B. Engaging with support groups and counseling

9. B. Reconstructive surgery after mastectomy

10. C. Data privacy and security concerns

Chapter 12: Global Perspectives on Breast Cancer

12.1 Epidemiology and Variations Across Countries

Breast cancer is the most common cancer among women worldwide, affecting millions each year. However, the incidence, mortality rates, and survival outcomes of breast cancer vary significantly across different regions and countries. These variations are influenced by genetic, environmental, socio-economic factors, and access to healthcare services. Understanding the global epidemiology of breast cancer is crucial for developing targeted strategies for prevention, early detection, and treatment on an international scale.

Incidence Rates

- **High-Incidence Countries**: Western Europe, North America, and Australia have some of the highest incidence rates of breast cancer. These higher rates are partly attributed to lifestyle factors, reproductive patterns, and the widespread use of screening mammography, which increases detection.

- **Low-Incidence Countries**: Countries in Africa and Asia tend to have lower incidence rates, though these rates are increasing as these countries undergo economic development and adopt Western lifestyles.

Mortality Rates

- **Disparities in Mortality**: Despite having higher incidence rates, high-income countries generally have lower mortality rates due to better access to screening and advanced treatment options. Conversely, low- and middle-income countries (LMICs) often have higher mortality rates due to late-stage diagnosis and limited access to treatment.

Survival Outcomes

- **Survival Rates**: Survival rates for breast cancer have improved significantly in high-income countries, reaching over 80% in some regions. These improvements are less pronounced in LMICs, where survival rates can be significantly lower.

- **Factors Affecting Survival**: Early detection, access to effective treatment, and healthcare infrastructure are key factors that influence survival outcomes.

Socio-economic Factors and Access to Healthcare

- **Healthcare Access**: Access to healthcare services, including screening, diagnosis, and treatment facilities, is a significant determinant of breast cancer outcomes. In many LMICs, limited healthcare infrastructure and lack of affordable care contribute to poorer outcomes.

- **Cultural and Social Factors**: Cultural beliefs and social stigma can affect breast cancer awareness and attitudes towards seeking medical help. Education and awareness campaigns are crucial for encouraging early detection and treatment.

Global Initiatives

Several international initiatives aim to address the global burden of breast cancer:

- **World Health Organization (WHO)**: Implements programs focused on cancer prevention, early detection, and management in low-resource settings.

- **Global Breast Cancer Initiative**: Launched by WHO, this initiative aims to reduce global breast cancer mortality by 2.5% per year, preventing 2.5 million deaths by 2040.

- **Non-Governmental Organizations (NGOs)**: Many NGOs work internationally to provide education, resources, and support for breast cancer screening and treatment in underserved areas.

Conclusion

The global perspective on breast cancer highlights significant disparities in incidence, mortality, and survival outcomes across different regions and countries. Addressing these disparities requires a concerted effort from governments, international organizations, healthcare providers, and communities to improve access to education, screening, and treatment. Through global collaboration and targeted interventions, it is possible to reduce the impact of breast cancer worldwide and move towards more equitable health outcomes for all women.

12.2 Cultural Attitudes and Access to Care

Cultural attitudes towards breast cancer and healthcare significantly influence access to care and outcomes across different populations. Understanding and addressing these cultural factors is essential for effective breast cancer prevention, early detection, and treatment strategies globally.

Cultural Factors Influencing Breast Cancer Care

- **Stigma and Secrecy**: In many cultures, cancer diagnoses, especially breast cancer, are stigmatized, leading to secrecy and reluctance to seek medical help. This stigma can delay diagnosis and treatment, adversely affecting outcomes.

- **Gender Roles and Expectations**: Cultural expectations about gender roles may deter women from prioritizing their health or seeking care due to perceived responsibilities towards family and household.

- **Perceptions of Illness and Treatment**: Beliefs about illness causation, fatalism, and mistrust of medical interventions can influence attitudes towards screening and treatment. Traditional and alternative medicine practices may be preferred over conventional medical care in some cultures.

Access to Care

- **Economic Barriers**: The cost of healthcare services, including screening, diagnostic tests, and treatment, can be prohibitive for many, especially in low- and middle-income countries (LMICs) and among underserved populations in high-income countries.

- **Healthcare Infrastructure**: Limited healthcare infrastructure, including shortages of healthcare providers and facilities, especially in rural areas, impedes access to comprehensive breast cancer care.

- **Education and Awareness**: Lack of awareness about breast cancer symptoms, the importance of early detection, and available treatment options contributes to late-stage diagnoses.

Strategies to Overcome Cultural and Access Barriers

- **Culturally Sensitive Education and Outreach**: Tailoring education and outreach programs to address specific cultural beliefs and practices can improve awareness and encourage engagement with breast cancer care services.

- **Community-Based Interventions**: Involving community leaders, religious institutions, and local organizations in breast cancer awareness efforts can help reduce stigma and disseminate accurate information.

- **Enhancing Healthcare Access**: Implementing mobile clinics, telemedicine, and other innovative solutions can improve access to screening and care in remote or underserved areas.

- **Training and Capacity Building**: Investing in healthcare infrastructure and training for healthcare professionals, including specialists in oncology, radiology, and surgery, is crucial for improving access to quality care.

- **Financial Assistance Programs**: Establishing financial assistance and insurance programs can help reduce the economic burden of breast cancer treatment on patients and their families.

Conclusion

Cultural attitudes and access to care play significant roles in the global fight against breast cancer. Addressing these issues requires a multifaceted approach that includes cultural sensitivity, community engagement, investment in healthcare infrastructure, and initiatives to improve education and financial support. By understanding and addressing the unique needs and challenges of different populations, healthcare providers and policymakers can develop more effective strategies for breast cancer care, ultimately improving outcomes for women worldwide.

12.3 International Collaborations in Research

The fight against breast cancer is a global challenge that benefits significantly from international collaborations in research. These partnerships bring together diverse expertise, resources, and populations to advance our understanding of breast cancer and develop more effective prevention, detection, and treatment strategies. International collaborations can accelerate scientific progress, foster innovation, and facilitate the equitable distribution of research benefits across different regions and populations.

Benefits of International Collaborations

- **Diverse Genetic and Population Data**: Collaborations enable researchers to study breast cancer in diverse populations, enhancing the understanding of how genetic, environmental, and lifestyle factors contribute to cancer risk and treatment responses.

- **Shared Resources and Expertise**: Pooling resources, including specialized knowledge, technology, and funding, allows for more ambitious research projects and the leveraging of unique capabilities of partner institutions.

- **Standardization of Research Methods**: International projects can help standardize research methodologies, making studies more comparable and reliable, and facilitating the aggregation of data across studies.

- **Accelerated Drug Development and Clinical Trials**: Collaborative efforts can expedite the development and testing of new drugs and treatments by enabling multicenter clinical trials that recruit participants more quickly and efficiently.

- **Capacity Building**: Collaborations often include training and education components that build research capacity in low- and middle-income countries (LMICs), promoting sustainability and independence in cancer research.

Notable International Collaborations

- **The Breast Cancer Association Consortium (BCAC)**: An international group focused on identifying genetic susceptibility loci for breast cancer. BCAC pools data from many studies worldwide, enhancing the statistical power to detect genes associated with cancer risk.

- **Global Alliance for Genomics and Health (GA4GH)**: Works to create frameworks and standards to enable the sharing of genomic and health-related data for research, focusing on ensuring data sharing is responsible and beneficial to patients globally.

- **International Cancer Genome Consortium (ICGC)**: Aims to obtain a comprehensive description of genomic, transcriptomic, and epigenomic changes in 50 different tumor types and/or subtypes which are of clinical and societal importance across the globe.

Challenges and Considerations

- **Ethical and Regulatory Hurdles**: International collaborations must navigate complex ethical and regulatory landscapes, ensuring research complies with local laws and respects participant rights and cultural norms.

- **Data Sharing and Intellectual Property**: Agreements on data sharing, intellectual property, and publication rights are essential but can be challenging to negotiate, especially when projects involve multiple stakeholders from different sectors and countries.

- **Sustainability and Equity**: Ensuring that collaborations lead to sustainable improvements in global health and that benefits are equitably shared among all partner countries is a key concern.

Conclusion

International collaborations in breast cancer research represent a powerful approach to tackling the disease on a global scale. By combining resources, expertise, and data from around the world, these partnerships enhance our understanding of breast cancer and accelerate the development of new interventions. Despite the challenges, the potential rewards of these collaborations for global health are immense, offering hope for more effective treatments and improved outcomes for breast cancer patients worldwide.

12.4 Exercise: 10 MCQs with Answers at the End

Test your understanding of the global perspectives on breast cancer, covering epidemiology, cultural attitudes, international collaborations, and more. Check your answers at the end to see how well you grasp these concepts.

1. Breast cancer incidence rates are highest in:

   A. Sub-Saharan Africa

   B. North America and Western Europe

   C. South America

   D. Southeast Asia

2. A significant barrier to breast cancer care in low-income countries is:

   A. Over-reliance on traditional medicine

   B. High incidence rates

   C. Limited access to healthcare services

   D. Lack of public interest

3. International collaborations in breast cancer research help by:

   A. Focusing only on high-income countries

   B. Providing diverse genetic and population data

   C. Standardizing patient diets globally

   D. Limiting data sharing to protect national interests

4. Cultural stigma associated with breast cancer can lead to:

   A. Improved early detection rates

   B. Increased funding for research

   C. Delays in diagnosis and treatment

   D. Enhanced privacy protections

5. The Genetic Information Nondiscrimination Act (GINA) protects against discrimination based on:

   A. Income level

   B. Genetic information

   C. Education background

   D. Geographic location

6. High mortality rates from breast cancer in LMICs are primarily due to:

   A. Early detection through widespread screening

   B. Effective traditional treatments

C. Late-stage diagnosis and limited treatment access

D. Overpopulation

7. One goal of the Global Alliance for Genomics and Health (GA4GH) is to:

A. Decrease genetic research funding

B. Enable the sharing of genomic and health-related data

C. Standardize clinical treatments in all countries

D. Promote genetic discrimination

8. In breast cancer care, telemedicine can improve access by:

A. Requiring in-person visits for all treatments

B. Providing consultations and follow-up care remotely

C. Eliminating the need for doctors

D. Increasing healthcare costs

9. The Affordable Care Act (ACA) in the United States:

A. Prohibits coverage of breast cancer treatments

B. Allows denial of coverage based on pre-existing conditions

C. Ensures coverage cannot be denied based on pre-existing conditions

D. Mandates breast cancer screening for all age groups

10. Stigmatization of breast cancer in some cultures may result in:

A. Faster treatment initiation

B. More open discussions about health

C. Secrecy and reluctance to seek medical help

D. Uniform global screening practices

Answers:

1. B. North America and Western Europe

2. C. Limited access to healthcare services

3. B. Providing diverse genetic and population data

4. C. Delays in diagnosis and treatment

5. B. Genetic information

6. C. Late-stage diagnosis and limited treatment access

7. B. Enable the sharing of genomic and health-related data

8. B. Providing consultations and follow-up care remotely

9. C. Ensures coverage cannot be denied based on pre-existing conditions

10. C. Secrecy and reluctance to seek medical help

Chapter 13: Nutrition and Breast Cancer

13.1 The Impact of Diet on Breast Cancer Risk

Diet and nutrition play significant roles in the prevention and management of breast cancer. Research has increasingly pointed to the connection between dietary patterns and the risk of developing breast cancer, highlighting the importance of nutritional choices in overall cancer prevention strategies. Understanding how certain foods and dietary patterns influence breast cancer risk can empower individuals to make healthier choices that may reduce their risk.

Dietary Factors Associated with Breast Cancer Risk

- **Alcohol Consumption**: There is a well-established link between alcohol intake and an increased risk of breast cancer. The risk increases with the amount of alcohol consumed.

- **High-Fat Diets**: Some studies suggest that diets high in saturated fats (found in meats and dairy products) may increase breast cancer risk, although the evidence is not conclusive.

- **Red Meat and Processed Meats**: A diet high in red and processed meats has been associated with a higher risk of breast cancer, especially certain aggressive forms of the disease.

- **Fruits and Vegetables**: A diet rich in fruits and vegetables, which are high in antioxidants and fiber, may have a protective effect against breast cancer.

- **Soy and Phytoestrogens**: Foods containing phytoestrogens (plant-based estrogens), such as soy products, have been studied for their impact on breast cancer risk. Moderate consumption is generally considered safe, and some studies suggest it may have a protective effect, particularly in Asian populations.

Dietary Patterns and Breast Cancer Prevention

- **Mediterranean Diet**: This diet emphasizes fruits, vegetables, whole grains, fish, and healthy fats (such as olive oil). Studies have shown that adhering to a Mediterranean diet may reduce breast cancer risk, particularly postmenopausal breast cancer.

- **Plant-based Diets**: Diets focusing on plant-derived foods, with limited consumption of animal products, are associated with a lower risk of breast cancer. These diets are rich in fiber, vitamins, and phytochemicals that may help reduce cancer risk.

- **Weight Management**: Maintaining a healthy weight through a balanced diet and regular physical activity is important for reducing the risk of breast cancer, especially for postmenopausal women.

Nutrition After Breast Cancer Diagnosis

For individuals diagnosed with breast cancer, a healthy diet can support recovery, improve outcomes, and reduce the risk of recurrence. Nutrition recommendations include:

- **Balanced Diet**: Emphasizing whole foods, including a variety of fruits and vegetables, whole grains, lean proteins, and healthy fats.

- **Limiting Alcohol**: Reducing or avoiding alcohol consumption to lower the risk of recurrence.

- **Weight Management**: Achieving and maintaining a healthy weight through diet and physical activity.

Conclusion

The impact of diet on breast cancer risk underscores the importance of nutritional choices in cancer prevention and management. While no single food or diet can prevent cancer, adopting a healthy dietary pattern can contribute to a reduced risk of breast cancer and support overall health. Ongoing research continues to explore the complex relationships between diet, nutrition, and cancer, aiming to provide evidence-based dietary recommendations for reducing breast cancer risk and improving survivorship.

13.2 Nutritional Guidelines During Treatment

Proper nutrition during breast cancer treatment is crucial for maintaining strength, supporting the immune system, managing side effects, and promoting healing. The treatment phase can present unique nutritional challenges, including changes in appetite, taste alterations, and gastrointestinal symptoms, which can affect a patient's ability to consume and absorb nutrients. Here, we outline nutritional guidelines to support patients through their treatment journey.

Maintaining Adequate Nutrition

- **Energy Needs**: Cancer treatment can increase the body's energy needs. Consuming enough calories is important to maintain weight and support healing.

- **Protein**: Protein is essential for repair and recovery. High-quality protein sources include lean meats, fish, eggs, dairy products, legumes, and nuts.

- **Hydration**: Staying hydrated helps manage treatment side effects such as fatigue and constipation. Water, broth, and electrolyte-replenishing beverages can be beneficial.

Managing Side Effects through Nutrition

- **Nausea and Vomiting**: Eating small, frequent meals and avoiding greasy, spicy, or overly sweet foods can help. Ginger and peppermint are natural remedies that may alleviate nausea.

- **Taste Changes**: Experimenting with seasonings, marinades, and different food textures can help find foods that are appealing. Using plastic utensils can reduce metallic tastes.

- **Mouth Sores**: Soft, bland foods and those at room temperature can be more comfortable to eat. Avoiding acidic, spicy, or salty foods helps prevent irritation.

Special Diets and Considerations

- **Plant-Based Diets**: A diet rich in fruits, vegetables, whole grains, and legumes can provide vital nutrients and antioxidants. However, it's important to ensure adequate protein intake.

- **Supplements**: Discuss any supplements with your healthcare team, as some may interfere with treatment. Focus on obtaining nutrients from food first.

- **Special Nutritional Needs**: Some patients may require special diets or nutritional support, such as enteral feeding, if they are unable to meet their nutritional needs orally.

Nutritional Support and Resources

- **Dietitian Consultation**: Consulting a registered dietitian who specializes in oncology nutrition can provide personalized dietary advice and help address specific nutritional challenges.

- **Supportive Care Services**: Many cancer centers offer supportive care services, including nutrition counseling, cooking classes, and workshops that focus on nutrition during and after cancer treatment.

Conclusion

Nutritional care during breast cancer treatment is a vital component of comprehensive care. Addressing the nutritional challenges and side effects associated with treatment can significantly impact a patient's quality of life, treatment response, and overall outcomes. Tailored nutritional strategies, developed in consultation with healthcare providers and dietitians, can help ensure that patients receive the support they need to navigate their treatment journey successfully.

13.3 Supplements and Herbs: Help or Hype?

The use of dietary supplements and herbs has gained popularity among breast cancer patients seeking to complement their treatment and manage side effects. However, the effectiveness and safety of these substances can vary, and in some cases, they may interfere with conventional treatments. It's crucial to critically assess the evidence supporting their use and understand potential risks.

Evaluating the Evidence

- **Limited Research**: For many supplements and herbs, research on their efficacy and safety in breast cancer patients is limited or inconclusive. Some may have beneficial properties in theory or in vitro studies, but lack substantial clinical evidence.

- **Quality and Purity Concerns**: The dietary supplement industry is less tightly regulated than pharmaceuticals, leading to potential variability in product quality and purity. This variability can affect the supplement's safety and effectiveness.

Potential Benefits

- **Symptom Management**: Some supplements and herbs are used to alleviate specific treatment side effects. For example, ginger may help reduce nausea associated with chemotherapy, while glutamine is sometimes used to manage neuropathy.

- **Nutritional Support**: Supplements can be valuable in addressing nutritional deficiencies, especially when dietary intake is compromised. Vitamins D and B12, iron, and calcium are common supplements prescribed to meet nutritional needs.

Risks and Interactions

- **Interference with Treatment**: Certain supplements can interact with chemotherapy, radiation, and hormonal therapies, potentially reducing their effectiveness or increasing side effects. For instance, antioxidant supplements might interfere with the oxidative damage that chemotherapy aims to induce in cancer cells.

- **Hormonal Activity**: Some herbs and supplements, like black cohosh or phytoestrogen-containing products, can have estrogen-like effects, which may be contraindicated in hormone receptor-positive breast cancer.

Best Practices for Supplement Use

- **Consult Healthcare Providers**: Before starting any supplement or herb, discuss it with your oncologist, pharmacist, or a specialized dietitian. They can provide guidance based on the latest research and your specific treatment plan.

- **Disclose All Supplement Use**: Inform all healthcare providers about any supplements or herbs you're taking to ensure coordinated care and avoid interactions.

- **Choose Reputable Brands**: Opt for products from reputable manufacturers that adhere to good manufacturing practices (GMPs) and undergo third-party testing for quality and purity.

Conclusion

While supplements and herbs may offer benefits for managing side effects and nutritional deficiencies in breast cancer patients, their use should be approached with caution. The key to safely incorporating these products into cancer care is through open communication with healthcare providers, critical evaluation of the evidence, and careful selection of quality products. By prioritizing safety and evidence-based practice, patients can navigate the complex landscape of supplements and herbs more effectively.

13.4 Exercise: 10 MCQs with Answers at the End

Test your knowledge on the role of nutrition in breast cancer, covering the impact of diet, nutritional guidelines during treatment, and the use of supplements and herbs. Review your understanding and check the answers provided at the end.

1. High consumption of what substance is linked to an increased risk of breast cancer?

   A. Water

   B. Alcohol

   C. Green tea

   D. Fiber

2. Which diet is associated with a reduced risk of breast cancer?

A. High-fat diet

B. Mediterranean diet

C. Low-protein diet

D. High-sugar diet

3. What is a recommended practice to manage taste changes during breast cancer treatment?

A. Increase salt intake

B. Experiment with different seasonings

C. Only eat bland foods

D. Avoid drinking fluids

4. Why might supplements be used during breast cancer treatment?

A. To replace conventional treatments

B. To enhance the effects of chemotherapy

C. To address nutritional deficiencies

D. To increase energy levels only

5. What is a potential risk of using herbs and supplements without consulting a healthcare provider during breast cancer treatment?

A. Improved recovery

B. Interference with treatment effectiveness

C. Guaranteed safety

D. Enhanced emotional well-being

6. The Mediterranean diet emphasizes the consumption of:

A. Red meat

B. Fruits, vegetables, and healthy fats

C. Processed foods

D. Sugary snacks

7. Ginger may be helpful in managing:

A. Hair loss

B. Nausea

C. Bone density loss

D. Lymphedema

8. Regular physical activity for breast cancer survivors can aid in:

A. Increasing the risk of recurrence

B. Decreasing hormone regulation

C. Rebuilding strength and improving mood

D. Reducing the effectiveness of treatment

9. Antioxidant supplements during chemotherapy are:

A. Always recommended

B. Beneficial for all patients

C. Potentially interfering with treatment

D. Mandatory for recovery

10. A key nutritional consideration during breast cancer treatment is:

A. Avoiding all carbohydrates

B. Staying hydrated

C. Consuming a high-sugar diet

D. Limiting protein intake

Answers:

1. B. Alcohol

2. B. Mediterranean diet

3. B. Experiment with different seasonings

4. C. To address nutritional deficiencies

5. B. Interference with treatment effectiveness

6. B. Fruits, vegetables, and healthy fats

7. B. Nausea

8. C. Rebuilding strength and improving mood

9. C. Potentially interfering with treatment

10. B. Staying hydrated

Chapter 14: The Psychological Impact of Breast Cancer

14.1 Coping with Diagnosis and Treatment

The diagnosis of breast cancer can be a profound emotional shock, leading to a wide range of psychological responses. Fear, anxiety, sadness, and anger are common emotions faced by patients. The treatment phase, with its physical side effects and impact on daily life, can further compound these emotional challenges. Effective coping strategies are essential for navigating this journey, supporting mental health, and promoting overall well-being.

Understanding Emotional Responses

- **Initial Shock and Denial**: It's common to feel disbelief and denial upon first receiving a cancer diagnosis, as a way of psychologically buffering the immediate impact.

- **Anxiety and Fear**: Concerns about the future, treatment outcomes, physical appearance, and the possibility of recurrence are prevalent sources of anxiety.

- **Depression**: Feelings of sadness, hopelessness, or loss of interest in previously enjoyed activities can occur, necessitating professional support in some cases.

- **Anger and Frustration**: Anger towards the situation, healthcare system, or even friends and family who may not fully understand the patient's experience is also common.

Coping Strategies

- **Seek Support**: Engage with support groups, counselors, or psychologists who specialize in oncology. Sharing experiences with others who understand can be incredibly validating and relieving.

- **Stay Informed**: Understanding your diagnosis, treatment options, and what to expect can help reduce anxiety caused by uncertainty. However, it's important to seek information from reliable sources to avoid misinformation.

- **Practice Self-Care**: Engage in activities that promote relaxation and well-being, such as mindfulness, yoga, gentle exercise, or hobbies that bring joy.

- **Maintain Routine**: Keeping a semblance of your normal daily routine, as much as treatment allows, can provide a sense of stability and control.

- **Express Emotions**: Journaling, art, or talking with loved ones can be therapeutic ways to express and process emotions.

- **Consider Professional Help**: If feelings of anxiety or depression are overwhelming, seek help from mental health professionals. Medication or therapy can provide significant relief.

Support for Families and Caregivers

- **Education**: Understanding the patient's diagnosis and treatment can help families provide better support and cope with their own emotional responses.

- **Self-Care**: Caregivers also need to take care of their own mental and physical health. Joining caregiver support groups and seeking respite care can help manage stress.

Conclusion

Coping with the diagnosis and treatment of breast cancer is a deeply personal and ongoing process. Embracing a range of coping strategies and seeking support from healthcare professionals, loved ones, and peer groups can significantly impact managing the psychological impacts of breast cancer. Acknowledging and addressing these emotional challenges is a crucial part of comprehensive cancer care, supporting patients' journey towards healing and recovery.

14.2 Mental Health Support and Resources

Mental health is a critical component of comprehensive care for breast cancer patients. The emotional toll of diagnosis, treatment, and the journey to recovery necessitates accessible mental health support and resources. Recognizing the importance of psychological well-being, various services and programs are available to assist patients and their families in managing the psychological challenges associated with breast cancer.

Professional Mental Health Support

- **Oncology Social Workers**: Specialized in cancer care, oncology social workers provide emotional support, counseling, and assistance with navigating the healthcare system and accessing resources.

- **Psychologists and Psychiatrists**: These professionals can offer individualized therapy and, if necessary, medication management to address anxiety, depression, and other mental health conditions.

- **Psychiatric Oncology Services**: Some cancer centers have dedicated psychiatric oncology departments that integrate mental health care with cancer treatment, offering tailored support for patients and caregivers.

Support Groups and Peer Support

- **Breast Cancer Support Groups**: Led by healthcare professionals or peers, these groups offer a safe space for sharing experiences, feelings, and coping strategies with others who understand the breast cancer journey.

- **Online Forums and Communities**: Digital platforms provide accessible options for connecting with a supportive community, offering flexibility and anonymity for those who prefer it.

Educational Resources and Programs

- **Patient Education**: Understanding the disease, treatment options, and what to expect can alleviate some of the anxiety and help patients feel more in control of their journey.

- **Wellness and Lifestyle Programs**: Many organizations offer programs focused on nutrition, exercise, mindfulness, and other aspects of self-care that contribute to mental and physical well-being.

Holistic and Complementary Therapies

- **Mindfulness and Stress Reduction Programs**: Techniques such as meditation, yoga, and tai chi can help reduce stress and improve mental health.

- **Art and Music Therapy**: Creative therapies offer expressive outlets for emotions and have been shown to reduce symptoms of depression and anxiety.

Navigating Financial Stress

- **Financial Counseling**: Services provided by hospitals or cancer support organizations can help patients understand insurance coverage, access financial assistance programs, and manage the financial burden of cancer treatment.

Resources for Families and Caregivers

- **Caregiver Support Groups**: These groups provide emotional support and practical advice for those caring for loved ones with cancer.

- **Family Counseling**: Counseling services can help families navigate the emotional complexities of cancer, improving communication and coping strategies.

Conclusion

Mental health support is an integral part of the holistic care approach for breast cancer patients, addressing the emotional, psychological, and social aspects of the disease. By utilizing a range of support services and resources, patients and their families can find valuable assistance in coping with the challenges of breast cancer, fostering resilience and promoting overall well-being throughout the journey.

14.3 The Role of Support Groups and Counseling

Support groups and counseling services play a pivotal role in the emotional and psychological well-being of breast cancer patients and survivors. These resources provide vital spaces for individuals to share experiences, express emotions, and receive guidance, contributing significantly to coping strategies throughout the cancer journey.

Support Groups

- **Shared Experiences**: Being part of a group with individuals who have gone through similar experiences can reduce feelings of isolation, providing comfort in knowing others understand the journey.

- **Emotional Release**: Support groups offer a safe environment to express fears, frustrations, and hopes, facilitating emotional healing and stress reduction.

- **Practical Advice**: Members often share practical advice on managing side effects, navigating the healthcare system, and balancing cancer treatment with daily life, offering invaluable peer support.

- **Variety of Formats**: Support groups may vary in their structure, including face-to-face meetings, online forums, or telephone groups, making them accessible to individuals with different needs and preferences.

Counseling Services

- **Individualized Support**: Professional counselors or psychologists provide one-on-one support, tailored to the individual's specific emotional and psychological needs.

- **Coping Strategies**: Counseling can help develop effective coping mechanisms for dealing with anxiety, depression, and the stress associated with cancer diagnosis and treatment.

- **Family and Relationship Issues**: Counselors can assist with the challenges cancer poses to family dynamics and relationships, providing strategies for communication and support.

- **Survivorship and Future Planning**: Post-treatment, counseling can support adjustment to the "new normal," addressing fears of recurrence and helping with the reevaluation of life goals and priorities.

Finding the Right Support

- **Cancer Centers and Hospitals**: Many offer in-house support groups and counseling services as part of their comprehensive care for cancer patients.

- **Non-profit Organizations and Charities**: Organizations dedicated to breast cancer support often host support groups, workshops, and counseling services.

- **Online Resources**: Digital platforms and social media can connect individuals with online support communities and virtual counseling services.

- **Referrals from Healthcare Providers**: Oncologists, nurses, and social workers can recommend reputable support groups and professional counseling services.

The Importance of Support Networks

- **Building a Support Network**: Engaging with support groups and counseling services can help build a broader support network, encompassing healthcare professionals, family, friends, and peers.

- **Holistic Care**: Addressing the psychological and emotional aspects of breast cancer is as crucial as managing the physical aspects, emphasizing the importance of holistic care.

Conclusion

Support groups and counseling play an essential role in the comprehensive care of breast cancer patients, offering emotional support, practical advice, and coping strategies. These resources empower patients and survivors to navigate their journeys with resilience, ensuring they do not face the challenges of breast cancer alone.

14.4 Exercise: 10 MCQs with Answers at the End

Test your understanding of the psychological impact of breast cancer, including coping mechanisms, mental health support, and the benefits of support groups and counseling. Verify your knowledge and check the answers provided at the end.

1. What is a common initial emotional response to a breast cancer diagnosis?

   A. Indifference

   B. Immediate acceptance

   C. Shock and denial

   D. Immediate action planning

2. Which of the following is a benefit of support groups for breast cancer patients?

   A. Reduced need for medical treatment

   B. Opportunity to share experiences and receive peer support

   C. Guaranteed privacy of shared information

   D. Financial assistance for all members

3. One-on-one counseling for breast cancer patients can specifically help with:

A. Providing medical treatment

B. Developing coping strategies for emotional challenges

C. Offering legal advice on healthcare rights

D. Organizing fundraising events

4. Anxiety and fear during breast cancer treatment can be alleviated by:

A. Avoiding information about the disease

B. Staying informed and understanding treatment options

C. Completely isolating oneself from support systems

D. Focusing solely on potential negative outcomes

5. Coping with the side effects of breast cancer treatment can be aided by:

A. Ignoring the side effects until they resolve on their own

B. Engaging in physical activities within personal limits

C. Refusing to discuss side effects with healthcare providers

D. Avoiding any form of emotional expression

6. Which of the following is NOT a role of oncology social workers?

A. Performing surgery

B. Providing emotional support and counseling

C. Assisting with navigating the healthcare system

D. Helping access resources and services

7. Creative therapies, such as art and music therapy, can help breast cancer patients by:

A. Replacing conventional cancer treatments

B. Providing a means of expression and reducing stress

C. Teaching patients about the biology of cancer

D. Acting as the primary form of emotional support

8. The role of nutritional counseling in breast cancer care includes:

A. Prescribing medications for treatment

B. Advising on diet to support overall health and manage treatment side effects

C. Conducting surgery and radiation therapy

D. Providing legal counsel on patient rights

9. Mindfulness and meditation can benefit breast cancer patients by:

   A. Serving as a cure for cancer

   B. Reducing stress and improving emotional well-being

   C. Increasing the effectiveness of chemotherapy

   D. Eliminating the need for follow-up care

10. Caregiver support groups are important because:

   A. They eliminate the need for professional healthcare services

   B. Caregivers do not experience stress or emotional challenges

   C. They provide emotional support and practical advice for caregivers

   D. Only caregivers are allowed to make treatment decisions for patients

Answers:

1. C. Shock and denial

2. B. Opportunity to share experiences and receive peer support

3. B. Developing coping strategies for emotional challenges

4. B. Staying informed and understanding treatment options

5. B. Engaging in physical activities within personal limits

6. A. Performing surgery

7. B. Providing a means of expression and reducing stress

8. B. Advising on diet to support overall health and manage treatment side effects

9. B. Reducing stress and improving emotional well-being

10. C. They provide emotional support and practical advice for caregivers

Chapter 15: Looking to the Future

15.1 New Frontiers in Treatment

The landscape of breast cancer treatment is evolving rapidly, with ongoing research and technological advancements opening new frontiers in the fight against this disease. Innovations in targeted therapies, immunotherapy, precision medicine, and minimally invasive surgical techniques are transforming the approach to breast cancer care, offering hope for more effective treatments with fewer side effects.

Targeted Therapies

- **Expanding Targets**: Beyond HER2 and hormone receptors, researchers are identifying new molecular targets for breast cancer, such as PI3K inhibitors and CDK4/6 inhibitors, which offer more personalized treatment options.

- **Combination Therapies**: Combining targeted therapies with other treatments, such as chemotherapy and immunotherapy, is showing promise in improving outcomes and overcoming resistance to treatment.

Immunotherapy

- **Checkpoint Inhibitors**: These drugs, which help the immune system recognize and attack cancer cells, are being explored in breast cancer, particularly for triple-negative breast cancer (TNBC) that lacks other targets for treatment.

- **Cancer Vaccines**: Research into vaccines that can prevent breast cancer recurrence, and potentially even prevent the disease from developing, is advancing.

Precision Medicine

- **Genetic and Genomic Testing**: Advances in genetic and genomic testing are enabling more precise identification of individual cancer characteristics, guiding the selection of the most effective treatments for each patient's specific type of breast cancer.

- **Liquid Biopsies**: This minimally invasive test, which detects cancer cells or DNA in the blood, is being explored for early detection, monitoring treatment response, and identifying changes in the cancer that may require a treatment adjustment.

Minimally Invasive Surgical Techniques

- **Oncoplastic Surgery**: This approach combines cancer surgery with plastic surgery techniques to remove cancer while preserving or reconstructing the breast's appearance.

- **Sentinel Lymph Node Biopsy**: A less invasive method for checking if breast cancer has spread to lymph nodes, reducing the risk of lymphedema.

Artificial Intelligence and Machine Learning

- **Diagnostic Tools**: AI is being used to improve the accuracy of breast cancer diagnosis through imaging analysis, potentially identifying subtle signs of cancer more effectively than traditional methods.

- **Treatment Personalization**: Machine learning algorithms can analyze vast amounts of data to predict treatment outcomes, helping to customize treatment plans to the individual patient.

Conclusion

The future of breast cancer treatment is bright, with new technologies and therapies on the horizon that promise to improve survival rates, reduce side effects, and enhance the quality of life for patients. Continued investment in research and a commitment to bringing these advancements from the laboratory to the clinic are essential for making these future treatments a reality. As we look forward to these developments, the hope for a cure and more effective management of breast cancer grows stronger.

15.2 Survivorship Care Plans

Survivorship care plans have become an essential component of post-treatment care for breast cancer survivors. These personalized plans outline a comprehensive strategy for monitoring and managing long-term health after completing breast cancer treatment. They serve as a roadmap for survivors, their families, and their healthcare providers, detailing follow-up care, potential late effects of treatment, lifestyle recommendations, and psychosocial support needs.

Components of a Survivorship Care Plan

- **Treatment Summary**: Details of the diagnosis, treatments received (such as surgery, chemotherapy, radiation, and hormonal therapy), and the treatment end date. This summary aids in the continuity of care and informs future healthcare providers of the survivor's medical history.

- **Follow-up Care Schedule**: Recommendations for follow-up visits, including the frequency and type of medical tests or imaging needed to monitor for signs of cancer recurrence or metastasis. It also outlines screenings for other cancers and ongoing assessments of treatment side effects.

- **Management of Long-term Side Effects**: Guidelines for addressing persistent or late-appearing side effects from treatment, such as lymphedema, neuropathy, cognitive changes, and menopausal symptoms. This may include referrals to specialists like physical therapists, neurologists, or endocrinologists.

- **Lifestyle Recommendations**: Evidence-based advice on nutrition, physical activity, smoking cessation, and alcohol consumption to support overall health and reduce the risk of cancer recurrence.

- **Emotional and Psychosocial Support**: Information on resources for mental health support, including counseling services, support groups, and survivorship programs, to help survivors cope with the emotional aftermath of cancer and its treatment.

- **Preventive Health Measures**: Recommendations for maintaining overall health, such as vaccinations, bone health evaluations, cardiovascular monitoring, and managing comorbid conditions.

- **Legal and Financial Resources**: Guidance on navigating insurance issues, employment rights, and accessing financial assistance programs to address the economic impact of cancer treatment.

Benefits of Survivorship Care Plans

- **Enhanced Coordination of Care**: Provides a clear post-treatment care pathway for survivors and their healthcare teams, ensuring that all providers are informed and aligned in their approach to ongoing care.

- **Empowerment**: Equips survivors with the knowledge and resources needed to take an active role in their health care and advocate for their needs.

- **Reduced Anxiety**: Helps alleviate concerns about the future by providing a structured plan for monitoring health and addressing potential issues proactively.

- **Improved Quality of Life**: By addressing physical, emotional, and social health comprehensively, survivorship care plans support a better quality of life post-treatment.

Conclusion

Survivorship care plans represent a key element in the transition from active treatment to long-term recovery, emphasizing the importance of ongoing care and support for breast cancer survivors. Tailored to each individual's unique experience and needs, these plans facilitate a holistic approach to survivorship, encouraging proactive health management and offering guidance for navigating life after breast cancer.

15.3 Advocacy and Raising Awareness

Advocacy and raising awareness are critical components in the fight against breast cancer. These efforts aim to increase public knowledge about breast cancer, influence policy and funding decisions, and support the needs and rights of patients and survivors. By engaging communities, policymakers, and healthcare providers, advocates work to improve cancer care, promote research, and reduce the burden of breast cancer worldwide.

Key Areas of Advocacy and Awareness

- **Education and Prevention**: Advocacy groups raise awareness about breast cancer risk factors, the importance of early detection through screening, and lifestyle changes that can reduce risk. Educational campaigns target diverse populations, emphasizing tailored messaging to reach different cultural and socio-economic groups.

- **Research Funding**: Advocates lobby for increased funding for breast cancer research, focusing on understanding the disease's causes, developing new treatments, and improving diagnostic tools. This includes support for both basic science research and clinical trials.

- **Patient Rights and Access to Care**: Efforts to ensure that all patients have access to high-quality cancer care, regardless of their financial situation, geographical location, or background. This includes advocating for policies that protect patients from discrimination and financial ruin due to medical expenses.

- **Support Services**: Highlighting the need for comprehensive support services, including mental health support, rehabilitation, and survivorship care, to address the full spectrum of patients' needs during and after treatment.

- **Global Initiatives**: International advocacy aims to address disparities in breast cancer outcomes and access to care in low- and middle-income countries. Collaborations between global health organizations, governments, and NGOs are crucial in these efforts.

Impact of Advocacy and Awareness

- **Policy Changes**: Advocacy can lead to significant policy changes, such as the enactment of laws that ensure coverage for mammograms and other screening tests, protect the rights of cancer patients in the workplace, and provide funding for cancer research and support services.

- **Increased Public Knowledge**: Awareness campaigns contribute to a better understanding of breast cancer, helping to destigmatize the disease and encouraging individuals to engage in preventive behaviors and seek medical care when necessary.

- **Community Support**: Awareness events and advocacy efforts foster a sense of community among patients, survivors, and their families, providing a network of support and shared experience.

- **Innovation and Progress**: By pushing for research funding and highlighting unmet needs in cancer care, advocacy drives innovation in treatment and support services, improving outcomes for breast cancer patients.

Conclusion

Advocacy and raising awareness about breast cancer are vital in promoting early detection, supporting research advancements, and ensuring equitable access to care. Through collective action and engagement, advocates play a key role in shaping policies, educating the public, and providing support to those affected by breast cancer, ultimately contributing to reduced mortality rates and improved quality of life for patients and survivors.

15.4 Exercise: 10 MCQs with Answers at the End

Gauge your understanding of the future directions in breast cancer treatment and care, including new treatments, survivorship care plans, advocacy, and raising awareness. Check your answers at the end to assess your knowledge.

1. New frontiers in breast cancer treatment include all EXCEPT:

A. Targeted therapies

B. Immunotherapy

C. Random treatment selection

D. Precision medicine

2. Survivorship care plans aim to:

A. Provide a detailed medical treatment plan only

B. Outline post-treatment follow-up care and lifestyle recommendations

C. Discourage patients from seeking further medical advice

D. Focus solely on physical recovery

3. Advocacy and raising awareness in breast cancer primarily seek to:

A. Decrease public knowledge about the disease

B. Influence policy and funding decisions for better cancer care

C. Promote a single method of treatment for all patients

D. Limit access to new and innovative treatments

4. Immunotherapy works by:

A. Reducing the effectiveness of the immune system

B. Helping the immune system recognize and attack cancer cells

C. Completely replacing chemotherapy in all treatment plans

D. Targeting only non-cancerous cells

5. The main goal of precision medicine in breast cancer is to:

A. Offer a one-size-fits-all treatment approach

B. Tailor treatment based on the individual genetic makeup of the tumor

C. Avoid using modern diagnostic tools

D. Discourage personalized patient care

6. Liquid biopsies are used in breast cancer to:

   A. Replace all other forms of biopsy

   B. Detect cancer cells or DNA in the blood for early detection and monitoring

   C. Serve as the only tool for diagnosing breast cancer

   D. Increase the need for invasive surgical biopsies

7. Advocacy for increased research funding in breast cancer aims to:

   A. Reduce the overall budget for healthcare

   B. Support the development of new treatments and diagnostic tools

   C. Discourage collaboration among researchers

   D. Focus research solely on cosmetic outcomes

8. A key component of a survivorship care plan is:

   A. Advising against any form of physical activity

   B. Recommendations for follow-up visits and monitoring for recurrence

   C. Ignoring any emotional or psychological impact of cancer

   D. Ensuring patients return to their pre-cancer lifestyle immediately

9. The role of oncoplastic surgery in breast cancer treatment is to:

   A. Eliminate the need for radiation therapy

   B. Combine cancer removal with cosmetic or reconstructive techniques

   C. Focus on treatment without considering the aesthetic outcome

   D. Discourage patients from considering breast reconstruction

10. The use of artificial intelligence in breast cancer care includes:

   A. Decreasing the accuracy of diagnosis

   B. Improving the precision of treatment personalization

   C. Replacing the need for human doctors entirely

   D. Limiting the use of modern imaging technologies

Answers:

1. C. Random treatment selection

2. B. Outline post-treatment follow-up care and lifestyle recommendations

3. B. Influence policy and funding decisions for better cancer care

4. B. Helping the immune system recognize and attack cancer cells

5. B. Tailor treatment based on the individual genetic makeup of the tumor

6. B. Detect cancer cells or DNA in the blood for early detection and monitoring

7. B. Support the development of new treatments and diagnostic tools

8. B. Recommendations for follow-up visits and monitoring for recurrence

9. B. Combine cancer removal with cosmetic or reconstructive techniques

10. B. Improving the precision of treatment personalization

Conclusion

As we conclude our exploration of breast cancer, it's evident that this journey encompasses a wide array of topics, from understanding the basics of the disease, navigating treatment options, coping with psychological impacts, to engaging in advocacy and looking forward to new frontiers in care and treatment. Each chapter has shed light on the complexities and challenges faced by individuals affected by breast cancer, while also highlighting the progress and hope that continue to evolve in the field.

Breast cancer, being the most common cancer among women worldwide, demands our attention and action—whether it's through research, clinical care, support services, or public advocacy. The advancements in targeted therapies, immunotherapy, precision medicine, and supportive care underscore the progress being made, yet the journey doesn't stop here. Ongoing research, increased funding, and global collaboration are essential to further improve outcomes, enhance quality of life for patients and survivors, and ultimately, move closer to a cure.

The role of patient advocacy and awareness cannot be overstated, as these efforts drive policy changes, increase funding for research, and ensure that those affected by breast cancer have access to the care and support they need. Empowering patients, survivors, and their families with knowledge and resources is crucial for navigating the breast cancer journey.

This comprehensive exploration of breast cancer underlines the importance of a multidisciplinary approach to care, incorporating medical treatment, psychological support, and lifestyle considerations. It highlights the necessity of individualized care plans that address the unique needs of each person affected by breast cancer.

As we look to the future, let's continue to support breast cancer research, advocate for patient rights, and provide support to those navigating this challenging journey. By working together—healthcare professionals, researchers, patients, survivors, and advocates—we can make a significant impact in the fight against breast cancer, offering hope and improving lives.

Thank you for engaging in this important conversation about breast cancer. May this knowledge empower you to take action, whether in your personal life, in supporting others, or in contributing to the global fight against this disease.

*The best way to thank an author is
to
write a review.*